Praise
MY JOURNAL

"I wish everyone could experience this process of awareness!"
—Wenke Andreae, Youth Coach at Leuker Leren Leren

*"**My Journal** helps you find peace and joy in life."*
—Dr. E.E. Maatman-Fleuren, NVO Generalist Educational Psychologist

"Maggie sees through it all: Your thoughts shape your sense of happiness."
—Rogier van Kralingen, author of Restart

"An accessible and valuable addition to the current guidance for girls."
—Elske Kolkman, Founder of Meisjescoaching Nederland (Girls Coaching Netherlands)

"For me, Maggie's Way was a real game-changer this year."
—Mariah Happe, author of the poetry collection, Puur

"A must-read for anyone who wants to improve their life!"
—Sander Koewe, Elite Trainers Group

"Offers young adults a highly accessible path to self-discovery."
—Guy Janssens, Organizational Architect at Management Assistance

"Maggie gives us all the tools we need to be true to ourselves and live our best lives."
—Rob Swymer, author of Surrender to Your Adversity

MY JOURNAL

MY JOURNAL

By Finding Yourself, You Find Your Happiness.

DREAM IT, BELIEVE IT, ACHIEVE IT.

START THE AWARENESS PROCESS
AND CREATE YOUR PERSONAL ROADMAP!

Maggie Maris

This publication is meant as a source of valuable information for the reader, however it is not meant as a substitute for direct expert assistance. If such level of assistance is required, the services of a competent professional should be sought.

Copyright © 2022, 2023 by Maggie's Way

All rights reserved. No part of this book may be reproduced or transmitted in any form or by any means, electronic or mechanical, including photocopying, recording, or any information storage and retrieval system, without permission in writing from the author.

ISBN: 978-1-6653-0679-9 - Paperback
ISBN: 978-1-6653-0680-5 - Hardcover

These ISBNs are the property of BookLogix for the express purpose of sales and distribution of this title. The content of this book is the property of the copyright holder only. BookLogix does not hold any ownership of the content of this book and is not liable in any way for the materials contained within. The views and opinions expressed in this book are the property of the Author/Copyright holder, and do not necessarily reflect those of BookLogix.

∞ This paper meets the requirements of ANSI/NISO Z39.48-1992 (Permanence of Paper)

Layout and design by Sacha Jeurissen, STUDIO ACHA
Translation by Helen Baldwin

1 1 1 4 2 3

☾ | ☀

*Your thoughts,
this beautiful booklet,
and you.*

DEAR YOU,	01
MY JOURNAL	04
TO KNOW	06
☉ BELIEVE IN CHANGE	10
☼ WHO AM I	50
❧ TAKING CARE OF YOURSELF	126
～ THE PLAN	192
A NOTE FROM MAGGIE	241
BOOKLIST	242
GET IN TOUCH	244
ACKNOWLEDGMENTS	246

Dear You,

I made this journal especially for you because I truly believe you can make yourself happy. The path to happiness lies in getting to know yourself and discovering what you need. Whether you are feeling happy or not, we all have our challenges, some more than others.

You will find it wonderful to work in this beautiful journal. The great thing is that it's all about you. It takes you on a personal journey and helps you get to know yourself so you can focus on doing what's best for you. As a result, you will naturally make better choices.

You will start to value yourself and learn to prioritize yourself too. Does it feel doable? It's an important and significant step that is crucial for your journey to happiness. You will realize that it's your life, not someone else's. You will learn to stand up for yourself, embrace who you are, and learn that you don't always have to conform to others' opinions. You will learn to treat yourself and others with respect. It may sound simple, but it's certainly not always easy.

"You gotta do the work"

All these things combined will help you enjoy what you do. You will achieve results and gain more self-confidence. You will begin to attract people who are compatible with you, people who also appreciate positivity.

Please, take time with your Journal—take as much time as you need. It's your process, so do it at your own pace. You will naturally sense when you've had enough for the moment. Decide for yourself when to pick up the thread again and dedicate attention to the most important person in your life—you.

Wrap life around you like a cozy scarf that is completely yours. By staying true to yourself and not comparing yourself to others, you will ultimately do the things that are right for you and who you are. This will bring you so much happiness and fulfillment!

Being completely yourself is my wish for you. My hope is that you discover a beautiful "true" you. A version of yourself that you may not have even known existed within you. You are unique and special, and I hope you come to realize and truly feel that. Feeling good about myself has been such a great gift. I felt liberated when I finally knew who I was, and I allowed myself to be true to me. I am still grateful for that decision every single day and you can experience that too. It would be fantastic if you inspire others to embark on this journey so that, together, we can make the world a little better.

I wish you a wonderful journey and don't forget to enjoy every moment along the way.

Lots of love,

Maggie

This is my journal

NAME

AGE

RESIDENCE

HOW WOULD YOU LIKE TO FEEL
AFTER COMPLETING THIS JOURNAL?

TO KNOW

How do I use My Journal*?*

This is your personal journal, belonging to no one else but you. That means you can use it however you want. The journal is divided into parts you can go through in order—and I do recommend following the order, as there is a common thread running through it. First, you'll prepare yourself for change, then you'll get to know yourself, next you'll learn to take care of yourself, and finally you'll set your changes in motion. When you know who you are, you have a better understanding of your needs and how to best take care of yourself. That's why I recommend filling out your journal from beginning to end. If it becomes overwhelming, take a break and come back to it later. Some information and exercises also need time to sink in. Some things require more thought to grasp, and that's perfectly fine! Put it to one side but continue when you feel the strength to do so. By completing this journal, you will notice changes in your thoughts, your life, and in your future.

What can you expect from this journal?

This journal is here to help you on your journey. It is a tool for finding happiness and making changes in your life. However, it's important to remember that a tool is not a magic solution, you still need to be willing and take action yourself. You need to be open to everything you will learn about yourself, your thoughts, and your environment.

You can expect this journal to give you new insights about yourself and your life. What you choose to do with those insights is up to you. To get the most out of this journal, it's important to apply what you learn to your daily life. *What do I think? What do I feel? What do I hear? What does this mean for me?* Expect this journal to provide you with a guide to get to know yourself, discover your dreams and needs, and hopefully find greater happiness in life!

Part 1 is about "believing in change." Do you believe you can change? Often, you may think you were "born this way" when it comes to a certain habit or characteristic and may even prefer to change it. During this part, you will become aware of your thoughts, behavior, and habits, and you will realize that you *can* change them. But only if you are open to it, that is! We are responsible for our own happiness. That's what part 1 is about. Do you believe you can change?

Part 2 is about "who are you" really and what you think of that. When you know yourself well, you know what's good for you. When you know what's good for you, you can meet your own needs. *What makes me happy? What are my dreams? What things bother me?* In this part, you will shift from your head to your heart and learn to listen to your intuition. The key is inside of you, the solution lies within yourself. Find your true self.

- **Part 3** is about "taking care of yourself." You now know what you need because you know who you are and what you want to change. Do you want to live a healthier life? Exercise more? Spend more time with friends or do you enjoy solitude? And why do you want these things? How do you stand up for yourself? These are all themes that will help you become the best version of yourself. You know who you are and what you want, now it's time to take action. It's about making choices that allow you to be who you want to be. This doesn't happen by itself.

"If nothing changes, nothing changes"

- **Part 4**: Let's get to work! During "the plan," you are ready to put everything into action. You believe that you can change, you know what you want to change, and how to do it while remaining mindful of who you are and what you need. At this point in the journal, you realize you can achieve anything as long as you believe in it. It's time to set goals and work toward them.

How do you feel at the end of this journey?

After completing this journal, you will have a better understanding of who you are and what you want. You will know what you want to change about the life you live today and about yourself. You genuinely believe that you can change. You have rediscovered the confidence in yourself, which you may not have realized you lost.

You will listen to your feelings and intuition and have the courage to follow them because you know you are right.

You know which goals to set, and you are confident you will achieve them, no matter how long it takes. You give yourself time and space to change. Ultimately, you will live a happier life because your thoughts are in order. As a result, you will experience less stress because you can give your feelings a place and put things into perspective. You also know which things make you happy and you make time for them.

Having fewer negative thoughts and experiencing a more pleasant and joyful feeling is the ultimate goal. I am confident that you can achieve this. Use this journal as a tool and commit yourself fully to it.

Part 1

Believe in change

- ***Believe in change . . .*** This is actually where it all begins. Do you believe you can change yourself? And what exactly does this mean? Before you realize you can change, it's important to become aware of your thoughts and behavior. Once you are conscious of them, you will realize that you have influence over them. If you don't know what you think or how you behave in certain moments, it's difficult to determine what you want to change.

  It all begins with self-awareness and observing how it affects you. In the beginning, it can be overwhelming to constantly pay attention to your thoughts and actions. You will then realize that we often have negative thoughts, whether about ourselves, others, the environment, or a situation. But it doesn't have to be this way! By engaging with this process, you will notice a shift in how you perceive yourself and the world. You have tremendous influence over your thoughts. They are not always true; they are just thoughts. Once you realize this, you will start feeling much better. We can literally choose how we think about ourselves and life, and often how we behave as well.

  For example, you are not inherently lazy, impatient, or a perfectionist. It is simply your behavior, and behavior can be changed. You are the one in control of yourself. How empowering is that?!

To do: Start by becoming aware of your thoughts.

What are the beliefs and thoughts you have throughout the day? (For example, judgments about others, negative thoughts about yourself, feelings of guilt?)

You are responsible for your own happiness. Unfortunately, we cannot blame others for it. Blaming others is something we often do, which is quite normal. However, at some point, you realize that by examining your actions and how you do things, you can exert influence, stand up for yourself, and feel much better. Blaming others is something we will delve into further in part 3.

To do: Causes of your emotions/feelings.

What do you think, is the cause of your life not going the way you want it to? Is it something or someone? Feel free to write down as much as you want.

_____
_____
_____
_____
_____
_____
_____
_____
_____
_____
_____
_____
_____

It's great to have your daily thoughts organized and to understand that you have influence over your thinking, but how do you get there and how do you do it?

You are initiating your process of self-awareness by writing down your daily thoughts. In the beginning, it can feel overwhelming, but it is an important part of your journey. Everyone can do this, but the key is to go at your own pace. You will notice that we are often inclined to think negative things, including about ourselves. What happens to you when you realize this? And what thoughts about yourself would you like to change?

To do: Your thoughts and beliefs are changing.

What beliefs/thoughts/perceptions about yourself and your life would you like to change? Think about the thoughts you wrote down earlier!

_____
_____
_____
_____
_____
_____
_____
_____
_____
_____
_____
_____

During part 1, the transition from a fixed mindset to a growth mindset is a crucial aspect. *"With a fixed mindset, you don't believe you can change, with a growth mindset you DO believe you can change"* (Carol Dweck, Mindset: The New Psychology of Success [New York: Ballantine Books, 2007]).

Ultimately, you want to shape your mindset in a way that allows you to change unwanted habits, thoughts, or behavioral traits. If nothing changes, nothing changes. Ask yourself the question: Do I want to change? What do I need in order to change?

Achieving your dreams and making significant changes in your life can only happen if you change yourself first. And you can! Your brain has the capacity to develop throughout your entire life. However, many people believe that change is impossible or too difficult. Does that apply to you as well? If so, you may have a fixed mindset rather than a growth mindset. It's important to change your mindset first in order to live the life of your dreams.

Everyone is born with a growth mindset. As children, we see opportunities and possibilities in every situation. A good example of this is the quote from Pippi Longstocking, "I have never tried that before, so I think I should definitely be able to do it."

A fixed mindset develops later in life, often influenced by negative experiences or criticism. You start believing that personal growth is dependent on talent, you often see obstacles and prefer to stay within your comfort zone.

The problem with a fixed mindset is that it often leads to a self-fulfilling prophecy. You believe that you cannot do something, and as a result, you don't make an effort to learn it. The outcome: your negative belief about yourself is confirmed, and your life remains the same. With a growth mindset, you can turn the self-fulfilling prophecy in your favor. You strongly believe that you can learn something, and you make every effort to improve. The result? Personal growth and development!

The connection with mindset is something that Dr. Carol Dweck (*Mindset*, 2007) discovered. Children with a growth mindset perform much better than children with a fixed mindset. This is because children with a growth mindset believe that they can become smarter. They focus on their personal development, are not afraid of hard work, and see failure as a natural part of the learning process.

On the other hand, children with a fixed mindset believe that their intelligence is, well, fixed. They focus on proving their intelligence or hiding any perceived deficiencies. They fear the judgment of others and avoid situations where they might fail. Although this research is about children, it applies to people of all ages. Thanks to the neuroplasticity of your brain, you can continue to develop throughout your life. However, this can only happen if you believe in your own ability to do so.

To do: Believe in change and growth.

When you change and grow in a positive way, you become better at something. As you improve, you naturally find it more enjoyable.

How do you feel about change and growth?
_____
_____
_____

Do you believe that you can do this?
_____
_____
_____
_____

In which situations have you experienced personal growth?
_____
_____
_____
_____
_____

Now that you understand why a growth mindset is necessary in order to change yourself and achieve your goals, it's time to let go of your fixed mindset. This process takes time and involves ups and downs. It starts with the firm belief that your life doesn't have to just go along as it is. You can take control and achieve almost anything you want. It's crucial to know why you want to change because strong intrinsic motivation sends a message to your brain to take action. Only then will you encounter the stimulating environments and experiences necessary for this phase of your personal development. Only then will you move closer to living the life of your dreams.

To do: Why do you want to change?

Do you still remember what you wrote down that you want to change? Why do you want to change it?

_____
_____
_____
_____
_____
_____
_____
_____
_____

FIXED MINDSET		GROWTH MINDSET
Shunning challenges	→	*Seeing challenges as fun*
Giving up	→	*Continue*
Seeing effort as futile	→	*Seeing effort as a path*
Not listening to feedback	→	*Learning from*
Feeling threatened at the success of others	→	*Learning from the success of others*

To do: Apply the growth mindset to your thoughts.

How do I turn these negative thoughts into something positive?

I overslept this morning

↓

I am starting my day today extra rested!

↓

Next time, I'll put my phone away earlier, which will help me fall asleep sooner.

The next time I feel disappointed in myself for not exercising, I will change this thought to:

_____
_____
_____
_____
_____
_____

Next time, I will:

_____
_____
_____
_____
_____
_____

The next time I think I've had a bad day; I will change this thought to:

_____
_____
_____
_____
_____
_____

Next time, I will:

_____
_____
_____
_____
_____
_____
_____

The next time I feel frustrated that I haven't completed my to-do list, I will change this thought to:

_____
_____
_____
_____
_____
_____

Next time, I will:

_____
_____
_____
_____
_____
_____

Having negative thoughts is not a problem; it happens to everyone. But now that you're on your way to developing a growth mindset, it's important to transform these negative thoughts into something positive. This doesn't mean you should justify certain behaviors, but rather think about how you can maintain a positive outlook toward yourself and how you can do things differently next time. Not every day is equally enjoyable, sometimes you need to take a break and do something "unproductive," your to-do list will never truly be completed, and occasionally going off track on weekends is part of life. It's about how you approach these situations with a positive mindset. The choice is entirely yours.

These choices will become easier for you over time. It's a process that requires practice before you become better at it. You'll start enjoying it more and more because getting better at something is always enjoyable.

Wanting to grow, wanting to learn, wanting to improve, having a growth mindset, and enjoying it all are the foundations of a great life.

Never stop learning, be open.

If **you** put your mind to something you can achieve **anything** you want.

To do: Make choices.

Now you know that your thoughts and beliefs are choices. Which thoughts do you choose?

This is how I want to think about myself:

_____
_____
_____

This is how I want to think about the people around me:

_____
_____
_____

This is how I want to think about the design of my life:

_____
_____
_____

This is how I want to think about managing my time:

_____
_____
_____

This is how I want to take care of myself:

_____
_____
_____

This is how I want to feel:

_____
_____
_____

You are getting a clearer picture of what you want to change and how you want to organize your life. This brings about change. Changes require initial effort, but eventually become effortless.

This is explained in the following model:

unconscious	→	*incompetent*
conscious	→	*incompetent*
conscious	→	*competent*
unconscious	→	*competent*

In the first stage, you are not aware that you lack a certain skill or ability. You are unaware that your behavior is not effective in a specific situation. You are unconsciously incompetent.

You can become aware on your own that you lack something or need to learn something new, or someone else can point it out to you. When this happens, you enter the second stage, which is being consciously incompetent: you are aware that you lack something and need to learn. However, you may not know exactly how or what to learn yet.

If you actively seek to acquire the desired knowledge, skills, or competencies, you enter the third stage: consciously competent. You are consciously engaged in acquiring the desired knowledge, skills, or competencies to become "competent."

Practice makes perfect, and when you demonstrate new knowledge, skills, or competencies without being consciously aware of it, you become unconsciously competent. You are no longer actively engaged in the new knowledge, no longer consciously thinking about it, but rather, you effortlessly demonstrate it without consciously trying.

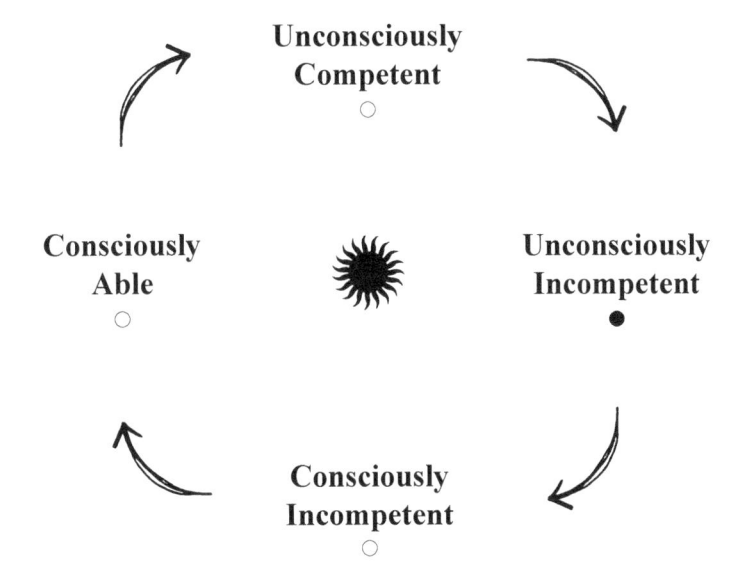

Unconsciously Competent

Unconsciously Incompetent

Consciously Able

Consciously Incompetent

To do: What doesn't come naturally yet?

You can't expect every change to happen effortlessly. In fact, change is always difficult, and it requires perseverance to turn it into a habit, such as developing healthy habits. What can work in your favor is knowing your weaknesses. If you're aware of what you struggle with, you also know where you need to put in extra effort. This will be further explored in part 2, but for now:

Where do I need extra motivation? (For example: exercising, getting out of bed, eating healthy, etc.)

_____
_____
_____

In which situations do you think: "I can't do it?"

_____
_____
_____

Which change(s) do you think you will have the most difficulty with, and why?

_____
_____
_____

A very important question is how you plan to stay motivated and disciplined. What will be your driving force?

_____

_____

_____

_____

During one of the previous to-dos, you tried to transform negative thoughts into something positive. With this to-do, you're going a step further. You'll transform your own thoughts, which you are becoming more mindful of, into something positive. While working toward your set goals and following your created plan, you will undoubtedly encounter setbacks. But don't let them discourage you! If your plan didn't work out perfectly one week, you have the next week to try again. It's never perfect, remember that. Focus on what you have already accomplished.

Take a moment to reflect on the negative thoughts that arise throughout your day and consider how useless they are in achieving your goals. Bringing yourself down will never take you where you want to be.

Think about how you can transform certain thoughts into something positive when they arise again, in order to not slow your own progress.

To do: Change your own thoughts.

For example, if you're thinking about your self-image, change your thoughts from "Throughout the day, I think I'm not good enough" to "I am as good as I am."

From:

_____
_____

To:

_____
_____

✦

From:

_____
_____

To:

_____
_____

From:

_____
_____

To:

_____
_____

✧

From:

_____
_____

To:

_____
_____

Let's go back to the fixed mindset and the growth mindset. In a fixed mindset, people believe that they are naturally skilled at certain things and that they cannot learn much more. In a growth mindset, people believe that they can continue to learn and grow throughout their entire lives because they keep trying and practicing. They are interested in things and ask questions. When you ask questions, you are learning and therefore growing. Life is always in motion for them because they are open to change and focus on what is possible.

Think in possibilities.

Simply put: Our way of thinking shapes our beliefs about achieving something.

We actually have influence over all the thoughts we have and our mindset! This can be a strange realization at first. You might think, "I've been doing or thinking this way my whole life, so it must be true. It's fixed." But the fact that you've been doing something a certain way your whole life is simply a matter of habit. And just like any habit, it can be unlearned and changed.

This is purely mindset.

Our mindset determines whether we believe we can change and grow . . . or not.

So, how do you train your mindset?

To do: Train your mindset. Here are seven mindset exercises that can help you develop a positive/growth mindset.

Focus on the positive things and on how you want your life to look. What is positive at this moment?

_____
_____
_____
_____

Accept what is currently in your life and be grateful. What are you grateful for?

_____
_____
_____
_____

Take responsibility for your life. What are you going to do to change your life?

_____
_____
_____
_____

Surround yourself with positivity and inspiration. Where will you find inspiration to achieve your goals?

___

Stop comparing yourself to others. How will you prevent yourself from doing this?

___

Eliminate all negativity. Which negative thought will you permanently remove from your mind?

_____
_____
_____
_____
_____

Discover who you are and what you want. This is a difficult question. We will delve into this further in a later part. If you'd like, you can try to put it into words here.

Who are you and what do you want in this life? What would you like to achieve?

_____
_____
_____
_____
_____
_____
_____

Do you remember when we talked about the "unconscious competence" model? In part 1, you were "unconsciously incompetent." You didn't know that you had no control over your own thoughts and were unaware of the fact that you could change. During part 1, you became "consciously incompetent." You discovered there are so many things you still don't know about your actions and their influence.

You will find out during part 2 that the goal is to become "unconsciously competent" and apply all the wonderful things you learn in your journal to your life without consciously thinking about it.

This is a long road with many bumps, but it is also a very beautiful adventure.

What did you think of part 1 so far?

_____
_____
_____
_____
_____
_____

To do: Summarize part 1.

After part 1, I have a better understanding of my daily thoughts, which mainly revolve around:

_____
_____
_____
_____

After part 1, I know **what** I want to change:

_____
_____
_____
_____
_____

After part 1, I know **how** I am going to change:

_____
_____
_____
_____
_____

After part 1, I feel:

_____
_____
_____
_____

Treat yourself with respect and love.
The rest will follow!

You have completed part 1. Well done! Are you proud of yourself? Purchasing this book and getting started with it is an accomplishment in itself, and you have every right to be proud. Keep going, as it will only get more enjoyable. After part 1, you will be open to change, and that is the beginning of your new life.

REPEAT AFTER ME:

✦ *I am ready to change my life.*

✦ *I believe that I can change.*

✦ *I believe in myself, and I am motivated to make it succeed.*

✦ *I am open to learning new things about myself.*

✦ *I accept that change doesn't come automatically and that I have to work hard for it.*

✦ *I don't blame others for my circumstances.*

✦ *I know that change doesn't happen automatically.*

Which emotions do you feel after part 1?
Circle, cross out, highlight, or add any that apply to you.

Motivated

Strong

Positive

CONFIDENT

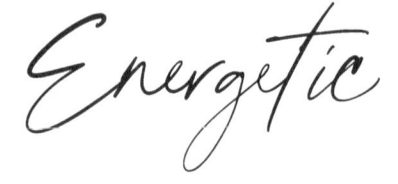

Energetic

RELIEVED

Proud

Touched

Happy

EMOTIONAL

Sad

Room for thought

✧ *Gratitude* ✧

Three things I am grateful for:

_____
_____
_____

Three things I am looking forward to or that were fun today:

_____
_____
_____

Three positive affirmations:

_____
_____
_____

Rate your mood

☆ ☆ ☆ ☆ ☆

✧ *Gratitude* ✧

Three things I am grateful for:

_____
_____
_____

Three things I am looking forward to or that were fun today:

_____
_____
_____

Three positive affirmations:

_____
_____
_____

Rate your mood

☆ ☆ ☆ ☆ ☆

✧ *Gratitude* ✧

Three things I am grateful for:

_____
_____
_____

Three things I am looking forward to or that were fun today:

_____
_____
_____

Three positive affirmations:

_____
_____
_____

Rate your mood

☆ ☆ ☆ ☆ ☆

Gratitude
helps you to see what's there instead of what isn't.

Part 2

Who am I?

☼ ***Who am I?* . . .** During part 2, you will get to know yourself. In part 1, you examined your behavior and thoughts. But that's not who you are—that's how you act and think. You now know that you can change that. However, it's important to discover who you truly are, so you can understand the root of certain behaviors.

What brings you happiness? What are your dreams? When you know this, you will also have a better understanding of why you do certain things, and you will be one step closer to changing them.

But also: what are your qualities? What are you good at? When you know yourself, you know what is good for you. When you know what is good for you, you can provide that for yourself.

We will also explore what you worry about, how to let go of it, and how to discover what truly matters to you. Taking care of yourself is something we will discuss in part 3. How can you take care of yourself if you don't know what you need as an individual?

This "journey of self-discovery," as many call it, is fun and interesting. It allows you to focus on yourself, even if you're not accustomed to doing so. Are you ready to explore and discover yourself?

To do: My qualities.

Which qualities do I personally believe I have?

(For example: disciplined, driven, social, enthusiastic, organized, flexible, empathetic, positive, confident.)

_____
_____
_____
_____
_____
_____
_____
_____
_____
_____
_____
_____
_____
_____
_____

What qualities do others think I have?

_____
_____
_____
_____
_____
_____
_____

What qualities am I most proud of?

_____
_____
_____
_____
_____
_____
_____

Behavior is *how* you do something and not *who* you are. But did you know that a large part of how you behave can be explained by your inner nature?

Statements like "I'm not a morning person" don't have to be character traits. However, it does mean that you struggle with waking up in the morning. These are things you can change, provided you understand the reasons behind them. Did you go to bed too late? Did you drink too much caffeine? Were your children keeping you awake? Did you neglect self-care? Did you push yourself beyond your limits? It could be that, as a person, you need a lot of rest, but you don't act on it because you don't know yourself well enough yet. So you're not necessarily "not a morning person," you're not listening to yourself and not taking rest when you should. This is related to stimuli. You can also address this with a mindset shift but be careful not to exceed your limits! Be aware.

Now we are going to look at what things you do and what these things mean this is your behavior. I discovered for myself that I started procrastinating when I didn't feel like doing something. Sometimes it's good and necessary to persevere—in other words, sometimes you need a kick in the butt. Maybe you find yourself pleasing others a lot. It's often nice to help others, but are you doing it because you genuinely want to or because you're seeking validation? These are interesting things to explore and become aware of. In part 3, you will learn how to give validation to yourself.

To do: Get to know yourself.

Indicate whether the following statements are true or false.

PLEASER

I sometimes end up in unpleasant situations that I could have avoided by being honest.	*True / Not True*
I feel guilty when I disappoint someone.	*True / Not True*
I always prioritize others over myself.	*True / Not True*
I know how much time I need to set aside for myself and how much I can dedicate to others.	*True / Not True*
My mind is filled with other people's problems.	*True / Not True*
If someone asks for help, I often agree immediately.	*True / Not True*

ENTERTAINER

I feel that it's my responsibility to make others happy.	*True / Not True*
I feel uncomfortable when there is silence.	*True / Not True*
In group conversations, I am often the one who listens.	*True / Not True*
I often take on the task of organizing activities.	*True / Not True*
I prefer being alone rather than being around people.	*True / Not True*
My social battery drains relatively quickly.	*True / Not True*

SLACKER

I put the cap back on the toothpaste tube.   *True / Not True*

I leave empty milk cartons in the fridge.   *True / Not True*

When I plan to exercise, I almost always follow   *True / Not True*
through.

Once I'm on the couch, it's hard for me to get   *True / Not True*
up again.

I prefer biking over using a car or public trans-   *True / Not True*
portation.

                                                     True / Not True
In the morning, I hit the snooze button more
than twice.

PROCRASTINATOR

I immediately take out the trash bag when it's full.   *True / Not True*

I fold the laundry right away when it's dry and put it back in the closet.   *True / Not True*

I plan a major deadline well in advance and distribute the work over the remaining time.   *True / Not True*

I know how to prioritize tasks.   *True / Not True*

I am good at effectively managing my time.   *True / Not True*

I have a to-do list that I usually stick to.   *True / Not True*

You now have a better understanding of how you behave in certain situations. This also relates to whether you are introverted or extroverted, whether you are highly sensitive, or if you might be gifted.

INTROVERT/EXTROVERT

Introverted people are more inward-focused and tend to be calm and thoughtful. They may be more sensitive to external stimuli. On the other hand, extroverted people are more outward-focused. They gain energy from being around others and tend to seek social interaction. They are often more sociable, feel less hesitation in approaching others, and may be less prone to overthinking.

You might recognize aspects of both introversion and extroversion in yourself at different times. But if you had to categorize yourself, which box would you place yourself in?

To do: Introvert or extrovert? Where on the spectrum do you think you fall?

INTROVERT ——————————————— EXTROVERT

Why do you think this?

_____
_____
_____

HIGH SENSITIVITY

High sensitivity is innate. You have it for life, just like the color of your eyes or your skin type. You cannot become highly sensitive at a certain point if you were not before, and it does not disappear. However, you can become aware of your high sensitivity, learn to cope with it, and learn to recognize its advantages. At the same time, it is important to realize that highly sensitive people feel more and need more time to recover.

Rest is crucial because life is all about balance. If you don't get enough rest, there is a greater chance of getting overwhelmed and experiencing burnout-related symptoms. What I often see is that highly sensitive people are more prone to these issues because the thalamus, the brain's switchboard, has a lower threshold. They notice things less-sensitive individuals may overlook and need time to process all that information deeply.

To do: Gain insight into your sensitivity.

	Yes/No
Can you tolerate loud noises?	○ ○
Do you like soft things?	○ ○
Do you cut labels out of your clothes?	○ ○
Do you get dressed right away in the morning?	○ ○
Can you handle change well?	○ ○
Do you prioritize helping others before yourself?	○ ○
Can you enjoy the smallest things?	○ ○
Do you tend to overthink?	○ ○
Do you prefer staying silent rather than having a conflict?	○ ○
Can you handle scary or violent movies?	○ ○
Do you have an eye for detail?	○ ○
Are you empathetic?	○ ○
Are you intuitive?	○ ○
Do you self-reflect?	○ ○

This checklist gives you an insight into whether and how sensitive you are. At the end of this journal, you will find a QR code with more information and a comprehensive test. For an official diagnosis, consult a specialist.

GIFTED

Giftedness is a subject that is not well-known enough. Gifted individuals are different, think differently, and, as a result, are often more vulnerable. Many people have no idea about their own giftedness, which can lead to depression or other serious problems, such as thinking you are dumb or worthless your whole life. While, in reality, you are much smarter than others! It is crucial to learn how to deal with things like perfectionism, your own high standards, a strong sense of justice, and a critical attitude toward yourself—all traits associated with giftedness.

What is the conclusion of all this?

The most important thing is to understand how you are wired, why you do the things you do, and how that influences your life. It's exciting to delve deeper into this through research. It's also beautiful to realize that we are all so different! Embrace your qualities, don't see them as a diagnosis or handicap, but rather as a bonus that makes you unique.

You are special!

The question now is: Do you understand yourself? Do you realize that you act in certain ways in certain situations because of how you are wired? Everyone is different, needs different things, and has their own instruction manual. And yes, "normal"—what is that really? It doesn't really exist. Everyone is truly different.

If you know you are sensitive and, for example, need time to recover after receiving a lot of stimuli, you understand where certain actions come from.

For me, it was good to just stay home and not fill my evenings with plans. But what did I do? I did what others expected of me. I was a huge people-pleaser and wanted to make everyone happy. I didn't know myself well enough to know that I needed rest after a party or a long day of school or studying. If you don't know what's good for you, then who does?

Also, take a look at your emotions. See what they do to you and take the time to really acknowledge them. Emotions are meant to be felt; they are there for a reason. Do you dare to feel your emotions? And how aware are you of your own feelings?

To do: Deal with emotions.

When I feel overwhelmed, the best thing I can do is:

_____

_____

_____

If I feel sad and I don't know why, then I need:

_____

_____

_____

If I am afraid of something but I still want to push through, the best thing I can do is:

_____

_____

_____

If I have doubts about something and need to make a decision, it works for me to:

_____

_____

_____

If I am nervous about something and I want to calm myself down, the best thing I can do is:

_____
_____
_____

If I experience feelings of insecurity about whether others like me or not, it helps me to:

_____
_____
_____

If I'm not feeling well about myself, I find it comforting to:

_____
_____
_____

If I am dreading something, the best thing I can do is:

_____
_____
_____

A significant part of who you are is what brings you happiness. Do you know what makes you happy? Do you dare speak it? Or do you feel ashamed of certain things?

Once you know who you are and what makes you happy, you can better set boundaries and design your life in the best possible way. You can plan your days around it and create an environment that brings you complete happiness!

Simply making yourself happy with the smallest things!

We often forget what truly brings us joy in the hectic pace of the day. Let's go "back to the basics," even return to the child within yourself, and ask: What truly makes me happy?

Let's start with the basics. What are your favorites?

To do: *My favorites.*

What are my favorite colors?
___
___
___

What is my favorite drink?
___
___
___

What is my favorite food?
___
___
___

Who are my favorite people?

_____
_____
_____
_____
_____
_____

What is my favorite vacation destination?

_____
_____
_____
_____
_____
_____

What do I prefer to watch on TV?

What is my favorite book?

You're starting to have a better idea of what brings you joy. Great job! We're going to ensure the things that make you happy are incorporated into your daily life. After all, don't you want to make yourself happy every day? You have every right to do so—it's your life! Of course, some days are more enjoyable than others. The thought of "today is just not my day" will still come up, but now you know how to handle that thought. It's okay to have a down day. Most of the time, you'll feel better the next day. Perhaps your perfect day also includes less enjoyable tasks, such as things you have to do. But try to make them as enjoyable as possible for yourself and think about how you'll feel once you've accomplished them.

Your perfect day is a balance between necessary tasks (which you make as enjoyable as possible) and things you genuinely enjoy. By actively engaging in this balance, you're telling yourself, "I value myself." And you truly should! Sometimes, we forget that. When you start dedicating attention to yourself, you'll start feeling better and better.

Now, tell me, what does your ideal day look like?

To do: My perfect . . .

My perfect morning:

My perfect afternoon:

My perfect evening:

_____
_____
_____
_____
_____
_____
_____

My perfect workday:

_____
_____
_____
_____
_____
_____
_____

My perfect weekend day:

_____
_____
_____
_____
_____
_____
_____

My perfect vacation:

_____
_____
_____
_____
_____
_____
_____

My perfect relaxation day:

_____
_____
_____
_____
_____
_____
_____

My perfect self-care day:

_____
_____
_____
_____
_____
_____
_____

My perfect day with friends:

My perfect day with a partner:

The next time you have a wonderful afternoon, evening, or any moment for that matter, fully enjoy it! Do you ever pause and appreciate the pleasant moments you experience? Perhaps you should do it more often?

However, we must be cautious of perfectionism. The perfect picture is often all-encompassing, making it impossible to meet those expectations. When expectations are high, the disappointment can be equally significant if they are not met. When something goes wrong, it's important to realize that everything is already okay as it is. It's part of life. You learn and grow from every mistake you make or challenging situation you encounter.

Things unfold as they do, and sometimes it's good to take things with a grain of salt. Often, a creative solution emerges unexpectedly! Especially with a growth mindset.

Letting go is a valuable skill to learn. We often find ourselves worrying about things that aren't truly important, especially things over which we have no control. Eventually, you will come to realize this yourself.

Ask yourself the question: How much energy do these thoughts cost me? Do they bring me anything? Do I have time to dwell on them? Do they help me? Is this what I want? Keep your focus on your goals and minimize your involvement with unimportant aspects, such as talking about others, negative thoughts, insecurity, comparison, or jealousy. They're not worth your energy.

The perfect picture is not always realistic.

To do: Practice letting go. Let go and be in the present moment, because in the present moment, everything is always okay.

☀

Find a comfortable place to sit or go outside. Close your eyes, take four deep breaths into your belly, inhaling for four counts and exhaling for six counts.

Repeat this ten times or for as long as you find it enjoyable.

Now, listen to the sounds around you for twenty seconds.

Open your eyes and look around. How does it make you feel? Do you notice a difference? You are truly in the moment. Pay attention to what happens to you during this moment.

What do you feel? What do you experience? Is it pleasant?

☀

It's okay if you still have one hundred things on your to-do list.

It's okay if you don't respond to someone's message immediately.

It's okay if your room is sometimes a mess.

It's okay if things don't always go as planned.

It's okay if your inbox is never empty.

It's okay if the laundry is not always done.

It's okay if you sometimes feel down about yourself.

It's okay if you're still in the midst of your own process.

It's okay if change doesn't come easily.

It's okay if you have a bad day.

It's okay if you feel like giving up sometimes.

It's okay to feel sad or angry.

It's okay to let things be for a while.

It's okay to let go of things.

What is meant to be, will be.

We're talking about letting go and overthinking. Why do you overthink in the first place? Overthinking is excessively thinking about things that are not actually important. But if they're not important, why do you dwell on them so much? It may be because you struggle to filter out what is and isn't important, simply because there's so much to think about. It also tends to happen automatically. You can get completely lost in negative thoughts and create doomsday scenarios in your head that almost never become reality.

Thoughts are often not true at all. It often helps to put things into perspective and look at the bigger picture.

What do I find important?
Are those things truly important?
Will those things still be important in a few years?
If someone else had this problem or thought, would I consider it important too?
Do the thoughts I have help me with anything?
Would you like to take a break from your mind?
Would you like to focus on feeling rather than thinking?

These are questions you ask yourself when you find you're caught up in your thoughts and feel like you have many unnecessary thoughts. It's a shame because it leaves less space for positive thoughts! Worrying is something everyone does, some more than others. Highly sensitive individuals may tend to worry a bit more. If you find yourself worrying about something, try to figure out if the issue you're worrying about is truly important. Use the questions from the previous page as a guide.

If it is important enough, worrying still won't help; you need to solve the problem. So, start looking for a solution and ask for help from loved ones if needed.

Is it a significant problem?
Does thinking a lot about the problem help?
Can I solve it on my own, or do I need help?
Is it even possible to solve it?
If yes, how will I solve it?

With this approach, you are not avoiding the problem, nor are you overthinking it. Instead, you confront the problem by finding a solution. Think in terms of possibilities rather than problems. If what you're constantly thinking about is not a problem but more like fear, or if it's a problem beyond your control, there's often only one option left: letting go. Let go and focus on the present, as we discussed earlier. This can make a tremendous difference.

Do you know how much time you waste thinking about trivial things?

To do: Analyze your worrying.

What are the things you worry about? How important are those things to you really? Write them down and rate them on a scale of one to ten, where one is unimportant and ten is very important.

How do I come across to others?   *1* —— X —— *10*

———————————————   *1* ———— *10*

———————————————   *1* ———— *10*

———————————————   *1* ———— *10*

———————————————   *1* ———— *10*

———————————————   *1* ———— *10*

———————————————   *1* ———— *10*

———————————————   *1* ———— *10*

———————————————   *1* ———— *10*

———————————————   *1* ———— *10*

What do I find important? Because that's also nice to know! What things are important to you and why do you consider them important? Are there things you are proud of? Did you know that when someone makes a stupid remark, it says more about them than you? This person may be jealous or struggling with themselves. So it's nice to stay true to yourself. Meaning can be found in big things as well as in small things. Enjoying the little things can be very rewarding. Useful questions to discover what you find important are:

How do I want to be remembered in the future?

In what (big and small) things do I find meaning?

Do I genuinely find something important, or do I think so because someone else does?

Where do I prefer to invest my energy?

Reflect on the moments that hold value for you: "What do these moments say about the things I consider important?"

Do you choose the positive or negative?

DON'T WASTE YOUR TIME ON THINGS THAT ARE NOT IMPORTANT.

To do: What do I really find important?

Take photos throughout the week of all the moments that you find beautiful and enjoyable, at least one each day and preferably more! It can be your cup of coffee in the morning, a beautiful sunset, a nice outfit you or someone else is wearing, or a photo from a fun party. You can store the photos in a separate album on your phone or arrange them in a video each week. Alternatively, you can print them out and paste them into your journal. Whatever makes you happy!

Now you'll have a nice overview of things that are important to you, things you value, and simply things you enjoy.

Do you feel yourself becoming happier when you think about what truly brings you joy? And what about when you consider which things you should let go of? Perhaps there are still things you haven't written down or things that make you so happy you want to write them down again.

It's time for your own Happy List. Anything you can think of, as small or as big as you want, write it down.

An activity? A specific scent? A person? An object? You name it!

You can cut out the page or write it on another piece of paper. Then, you can hang your Happy List in a beautiful spot in your home, so you'll always be reminded of the things that bring you joy. By allowing yourself to enjoy these things, you make yourself a little bit happier every day.

MY HAPPY LIST

Often, when you know what you're good at, you also enjoy it. Perhaps you're hesitant to admit that you're skilled at something. Many people immediately think of talents, such as being good at a sport or singing. But you can keep it small as well.

For example, are you good at comforting or reassuring people? Are you a good listener or do you believe you have good social skills? Or do you have a distinct talent, like drawing or something else creative?

Often, you're also influenced by your environment. People have certain expectations of you. Parents, for instance, may want their children to pursue a higher education. But they question: Am I actually good at studying? Or do my talents lie elsewhere? Can I be true to myself? Do I feel good about it?

Another way in which your environment influences you is that you may stop paying attention to things you're good at because of what others think or due to other obstacles like money, time, or impracticality.

Later on in life, you often find yourself coming back to those things. You remember that you were good at them and that you enjoyed them. Why did you stop in the first place? When you do something from the heart, it doesn't feel like an effort, and it comes naturally. It's like being in a state of flow! You enter a flow of meaning and purpose, and that's where we all want to be. It brings immense joy!

To do: What am I good at and also enjoy doing?

SPORT

_____

_____

_____

_____

WORK

_____

_____

_____

_____

SOCIAL

_____

_____

_____

_____

CREATIVE

_____

_____

_____

_____

Work occupies a significant part of our lives. Regardless of how you look at it, money needs to be earned to meet basic needs. Some may need to work harder than others, but it is important for everyone to pursue their career dreams. Do something you enjoy! What have you always wanted to do? This, of course, varies for each individual. Nowadays, you see many people quitting their nine-to-five jobs to work from their laptops out in the warm country. They often encourage others to do the same. Whilst it's exciting, everyone has their own career dreams. It's perfectly fine if you do want a full-time office job. That's okay too.

What brings you happiness? That's what matters. Don't let the hustle culture drive you crazy. Look for what gives you energy. If your current job doesn't provide that, you can consider making changes. It's challenging, but it becomes easier when you know what you're good at! We discussed this in the previous "to do" item.

Did you write down any competencies under "work" in the previous task that you also enjoy? Use this knowledge to your advantage when exploring your career path.

What do I want? Or am I already content? It's truly a celebration to turn something you're good at and enjoy into your work. You get to make yourself happy every day and get paid for it!

The ideal situation.

"Do what you love."

As we discussed earlier in part 2, almost everything has its downsides, including work. The key is to make it as enjoyable as possible for yourself. If you're struggling with this, ask for help:

To do: My dream job.
This is my current job/work: [Please fill in your current job/work]

During the course of my work, I feel:

_____
_____
_____
_____

My strongest qualities in the workplace are:

_____
_____
_____
_____

If I could choose any type of work in the world, I would:

_____
_____
_____
_____

My ideal work situation would be:

_____
_____
_____
_____

Having an enjoyable job that provides challenges is necessary for feeling good and important, as well as receiving recognition for what you do. The feeling of personal and professional growth is crucial. If you find yourself going to work, studying, or engaging in any other daily activities reluctantly, something isn't right.

The more enjoyable your work is, the more you enter a state of flow without self-imposed or external pressure.

The more you enjoy your work, the less recovery time you'll need from it.

You now have a much better understanding of who you are and what makes you happy, what you enjoy doing, and what you're good at. That's already a lot of self-knowledge that you may not have had before. Isn't it wonderful? Unfortunately, life doesn't always go as we would like it to. Ideally, every day would be a "perfect day" as described in the previous task. However, our lives sometimes take unexpected turns, and there are situations where we have little or no control.

Things happen the way they happen. By accepting certain things, you save yourself a lot of worry. Don't misunderstand this: you still have control over your own life. But what if you start leading your life the way you want it, instead of letting your life lead you? Feel that you have control over your life, because you realize you have choices—choices you can make for yourself. Think in terms of possibilities, rather than problems. Ask yourself, what if I want to do something different from what I'm doing now? And what do I want? Once you realize that essentially anything is possible, that's when it becomes truly exciting.

Of course, you can come up with excuses for everything: "I don't have time because I have children" or "I don't have energy because I work too much." Do you recognize this within yourself?

What if you set aside these excuses, what do you long for in the depths of your being? Dare to dream and take action toward those dreams! Starting is challenging, but following through might be even more difficult. Do you want to lead your best life? *Dream big and put in the work*!

You can do it. Believe in yourself!

To do: How do your dreams look?

Where do you want to live in the future and with whom?

_____
_____
_____
_____
_____
_____
_____
_____

What do you want to earn your money doing? Think about your dream job that you described!

_____
_____
_____
_____
_____
_____
_____

What trips do you want to take? Where?

_____
_____
_____
_____
_____
_____
_____

What do you want to contribute to the world?

What do you want to do for others?

What do you want less of?

_____
_____
_____
_____
_____
_____
_____

What do you want more of?

_____
_____
_____
_____
_____
_____
_____

Describe your dream life once again, specifically using the answers you provided. And remember: dream big!

When it comes to pursuing your dreams, setbacks are inevitable. How do you handle them? What can you do when something goes completely wrong in your eyes? The most important thing is to acknowledge how something affects you and consider whether you immediately feel guilty about a setback. Even if you are "at fault" for something, it's important to remember that making a mistake wasn't your intention. We all make mistakes; it's a natural part of learning. You didn't do it on purpose, so there's no need to feel guilty, right?

If you don't feel guilty, what do you feel? Like you've failed? "Failure" is just a word in your mind. You're always doing your best. It hasn't worked out yet, but it will. If you still feel fear, disappointment, or even panic, it's okay to feel that way, but you can also let it go. It takes practice, but it will greatly help you. There is a solution to every problem. Don't blame yourself immediately; be kind to yourself.

Look at the cause of the problem: Can you do something about it? Yes? Then think about what you can do. No? Well, the answer speaks for itself:
Let it go.

Also, allow yourself to feel any emotions that arise. Cry when you're sad and even scream when you're frustrated or angry if necessary. However, don't let emotions take over. Determine how significant a setback truly is. Sometimes, life is "unfair." Fall down, get up, learn from it, and keep going. See it as a challenge, try not to take it too seriously—laugh about it, and think, *we'll find a solution for this too*. Some things just happen, and they make us more resilient.

To do: Setbacks.

What is the last setback you can remember?

_____
_____
_____
_____
_____
_____

How did you deal with it at that time?

Can you handle it better next time? If yes, how?

Do you have any regrets?

Will you ask for help next time? If yes, from whom? And how?

_____
_____
_____
_____

How did this setback make you feel? How did you feel afterward?

_____
_____
_____
_____

How did you allow these emotions to come in? Did it help?

_____
_____
_____
_____

Setbacks are part of our lives; they make us resilient. Your mental resilience determines how you deal with change, adversity, or negativity. The great thing is that mental resilience can be learned; it is a skill. Rob Swymer describes in his book, *Surrender to Your Adversity*, how to train the resilience muscle. The stronger it is, the easier it becomes to handle setbacks, so you can still maintain a positive outlook on life.

What are your pitfalls? When you know them, you can better manage them and see them as challenges.

To do: What are your pitfalls?

For example, a short attention span, impatience, etc.

_____

_____

_____

How do I personally deal with setbacks? I quickly switch gears when something cannot, may not, or does not work out. If that's the case, we go in a different direction. It's not a big deal. Sometimes it's unfortunate, so allow yourself to feel those emotions as well. Be open to help and feedback from others, so that it might work out next time. The people around you are there to support you, so let them in.

Also, don't take feedback too personally or see it as an attack. Do you feel like someone is judging you for who you are? Or is it not constructive feedback and just unkind? Realize that when someone says something unpleasant, it often says more about them than about you. This person may be in a bad mood, jealous, or tired. This is called projection: attributing (often negative) qualities or emotions to others so that we don't have to confront them ourselves. So, you can let that stay with the other person; it's not about you.

Be open to feedback, don't quickly perceive it as an attack, but rather take it in and grow from it. Be mindful of projection. Are you open to being coached?

To do: Are you open to feedback?

	Yes/No
I believe I can receive feedback well.	○ ○
When I receive feedback, I take action on it.	○ ○
I often perceive negative feedback as an attack.	○ ○
I know how to effectively work with feedback.	○ ○
If I make a mistake, I admit it.	○ ○
Asking for feedback is challenging for me.	○ ○
I often consider feedback to be helpful.	○ ○
My emotions overwhelm me when I receive feedback.	○ ○

Do you sometimes get stuck in setbacks or feel like everything is going wrong? It often isn't the case. It only seems that way because the negative aspects dominate, and you forget about the positive. If you dwell on a situation for too long and don't look beyond it, you may continue to feel stuck. By acknowledging out loud that you're getting caught up in a situation, you'll notice that you can step out of this negativity. Those emotions are natural and the last thing you should do is ignore them, so allow yourself to feel them. Then it's time to move forward and be realistic. Whatever you do, you will eventually overcome it.

Accept your setbacks, and in time, you'll look back on certain events and see how much you've learned from them. Unfortunately, this doesn't mean that setbacks won't occur in the future. But by following these points, we can leave them behind with peace of mind, close that chapter, and see them as lessons. Then you can refocus on what is going well.

To do: Look on the bright side.

What works well is creating a list of accomplishments, a "triumph" list. This way, you focus on the things that have succeeded (achieved). They can be small things too. You can hang this list somewhere or keep it on your phone. Every time you feel down about a setback, you can look at it and remind yourself how well you're doing. Allow yourself to feel proud in those moments.

MY TRIUMPH LIST

Back to the "unconscious incompetence" model for a moment. At this point, you are "consciously incompetent," but on your way to becoming "consciously competent." You are now much more aware of who you are, what you want, what you can do, and what you need. In part 3, you will learn how to take care of yourself so that you can take the step toward becoming consciously competent now that you know much more about yourself.

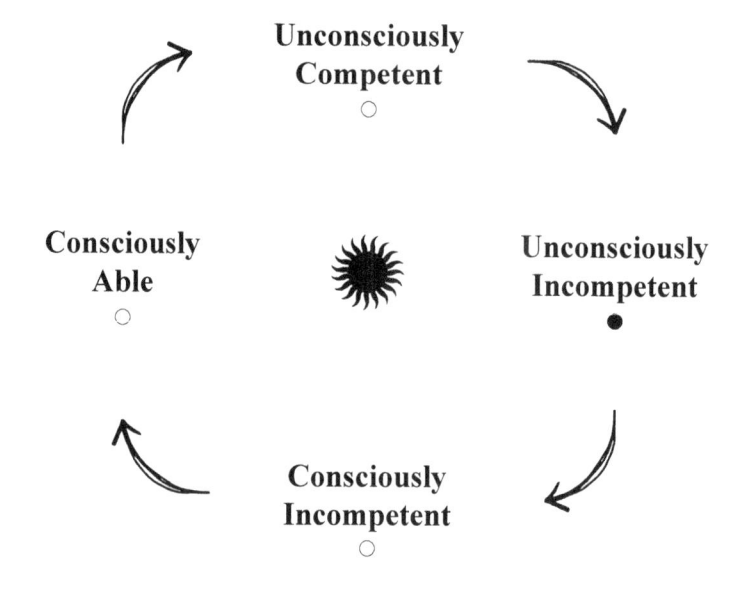

Unconsciously Competent

Consciously Able

Unconsciously Incompetent

Consciously Incompetent

To do: Summarize part 2.

After part 2, I have a better understanding of my core qualities, which include:

_____
_____
_____
_____
_____

After part 2, I know how sensitive I am, namely:

_____
_____
_____
_____
_____

After part 2, I know what makes me happy, namely:

_____
_____
_____
_____
_____

After part 2, I know what my strengths are, namely:

After part 2, I know what I tend to worry about the most, namely:

After part 2, I know what is truly important to me, namely:

After part 2, I know what my dreams are, namely:

_____
_____
_____
_____

After part 2, I know how to deal with setbacks, namely:

_____
_____
_____
_____

After part 2, I feel:

_____
_____
_____
_____

This concludes part 2! From my perspective, it was quite challenging, but also incredibly rewarding. As you go through each year, you will continue to rediscover yourself. Life experiences shape you, encounters with others offer new perspectives, insights emerge, and you grow older. When you discover what brings you joy and fulfillment, recognize your strengths, and identify your dreams. Prioritize yourself.

As a result, you start to believe in yourself, gain more self-confidence, and experience improved well-being. You now know who you are and consider yourself worthy of self-care because you understand your own needs. In part 3, we will delve deeper into this process.

You're already doing so well, don't forget that.

Keep going!

REPEAT AFTER ME:

- *I know who I am and what I need.*
- *I am perfect just the way I am.*
- *I know what brings me happiness.*
- *I will always advocate for my own interests.*
- *I dare to dream because I know I can achieve it.*
- *I am who I am, and others accept me for who I am.*
- *I know my strengths and areas for further development.*
- *I accept my flaws and do my best.*
- *I am proud of myself.*
- *I think about possibilities.*
- *I am open to coaching and guidance.*
- *I believe in myself.*
- *I love myself.*

Which emotions do you feel after part 2?
Circle, strike, highlight, or add the ones that apply to you.

Motivated

Strong

Positive

CONFIDENT

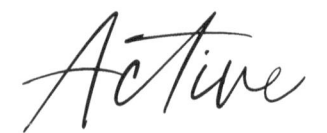

Active

RELIEVED

Proud

Touched

Happy

EMOTIONAL

Sad

Room for thought

✧ *Gratitude* ✧

Three things I am grateful for:

_____
_____
_____
_____

Three things I am looking forward to or that were fun today:

_____
_____
_____
_____

Three positive affirmations:

_____
_____
_____
_____

Rate your mood

☆ ☆ ☆ ☆ ☆

✧ *Gratitude* ✧

Three things I'm grateful for:

_____
_____
_____
_____

Three things I am looking forward to or that were fun today:

_____
_____
_____
_____

Three positive affirmations:

_____
_____
_____
_____

Rate your mood

☆ ☆ ☆ ☆ ☆

✦ *Gratitude* ✦

Three things I'm grateful for:

_____
_____
_____
_____

Three things I am looking forward to or that were fun today:

_____
_____
_____
_____

Three positive affirmations:

_____
_____
_____
_____

Rate your mood

☆ ☆ ☆ ☆ ☆

"It always seems impossible until it's done."

—Nelson Mandela

Part 3

Taking care of yourself

- ❧ ***Taking care of yourself . . .*** How do you take care of yourself? How do you know what you need? During part 2, you learned what brings you joy and what makes you happy. You also gained a better understanding of who you are as a person. In part 3, you will learn how to take care of yourself in different aspects of your life and take responsibility for it yourself. Everyone has control over it because we are responsible for our own happiness. Therefore, it is important to take good care of yourself, both physically and mentally.

Self-confidence and self-love start with taking care of yourself. After all, you take care of the people you love, don't you? You want the people around you, such as your friends, family, or children, to be well and happy. Why wouldn't you want the same for yourself? When you grant yourself the same care, you automatically start seeing yourself as important and deserving. Because you truly are. You deserve to be taken care of. Once you begin to realize this, your self-confidence receives a tremendous boost, and things start falling into place. At that moment, you dare to take control, stand up for yourself, and take responsibility for your own happiness. That's why it's incredibly important to take good care of yourself, both physically and mentally. In this way, you will also appreciate what your body does for you, and it will be able to do even more for you because you are taking better care of it!

How do you take care of your body and mind? In part 3, we will focus on the most important topics: nutrition, exercise, me-time, standing up for yourself, and facing your fears. Sometimes taking care of yourself also means doing things that you may be apprehensive about.

Taking care of yourself doesn't just mean pampering yourself, but being kind to yourself is the most important aspect. "Bad" self-care can also involve things like drinking too much alcohol at a party or indulging in unhealthy food while on vacation. However, sometimes indulging a little can make you very happy and be good for your mind.

Finding a good balance is what it's all about. Are you ready to start taking care of yourself?

☾

To do: Take care of myself.

Taking good care of myself means:

_____
_____
_____
_____

When I take good care of myself, I feel:

_____
_____
_____
_____

If I neglect self-care, it results in:

_____
_____
_____
_____

This is what I prefer to do to take care of my mental health:

_____
_____
_____
_____
_____
_____
_____
_____

This is what I prefer to do to take care of my physical health:

_____
_____
_____
_____
_____
_____
_____
_____

Nutrition

Everyone enjoys feeling good and confident. What I have noticed is that when you take good care of yourself, you easily become proud of yourself because you are giving yourself attention. Take the time to listen to your body as well. You are the only one who can truly feel what is good for you.

Nutrition is a significant part of this. Don't you deserve to eat well? By doing so, you will start feeling much better, both physically and mentally. When you eat healthily, you automatically feel more energetic because you will notice that certain foods give you energy while others make you feel tired. You may have never paid much attention to this because you have been eating in a certain way your whole life. You had sandwiches at school and meatballs at your grandparents' house.

But what if it can be different?

Our bodies are truly amazing. How wonderful is it to help that miracle by giving it the right things every day? One of the most crucial things that is often underestimated is hydration—in other words, drinking enough water. It is incredibly important to drink plenty of water every day (1.5/3L). Your cells need it to function properly. Of course, you also need the right vitamins and minerals. Eat an adequate amount of fruits, vegetables, nuts, and so on. Find your balance in this because going to extremes is never good. Be gentle with yourself, as only eating healthy every day is nearly impossible. Just pick up where you left off the next day. Being conscious of what you put in your mouth is already a significant step. Also, pay attention to your eating habits: take the time to prepare your meals, sit down while eating, and be mindful during your meals. Try to find enjoyment in it, be kind to yourself, and avoid emotional eating. You can do this!

To do: Have fun with recipes.

Fill in your favorite recipes! I've provided a few examples as a starting point.

Healthy breakfast recipes:

Oatmeal with plant-based milk, banana, and red fruits.

Plant-based yogurt, granola, and blueberries.

"Indulgent" breakfast recipes:

Healthy lunch recipes:

Avocado toast with cottage cheese, tomato, and chili flakes.

"Indulgent" lunch recipes:

Healthy dinner recipes:

Falafel bowl with quinoa, spinach, salsa, and hummus.

"Indulgent" dinner recipes:

I don't believe in strict diets because they often impose restrictions on oneself. I believe that each person should find their own path in determining what is good for them and what feels good in their stomach. Everyone is different, and each day is different.

How do you feel after eating certain foods? What does your body tell you? Did you really have a craving for it? Try to become more aware of what you truly desire. Often, your body actually needs exactly that. If you experience bloating or stomach pain after a particular meal, it's useful to figure out the cause.

Tip: You can also consider getting a food intolerance test! People who have trouble with dairy or gluten, for example, often discover it after a long time. The sooner you identify what your body can't tolerate, the better.

To do: Pick your meal.

Write down your all-time favorite recipes.

My all-time favorite meal:
_____
_____

My cheat meal:
_____
_____

Food that makes me feel good:
_____
_____

Food that makes me feel bad:
_____
_____

Something I don't like:

_____
_____
_____
_____

Something I would like to be able to make myself:

_____
_____
_____
_____

My go-to recipe:

_____
_____
_____
_____

If I were to create a three-course menu, it would consist of:

_____

_____

_____

_____

_____

_____

A good guideline to follow is the 80/20 rule. This means that you eat healthy 80 percent of the time and indulge in less healthy options 20 percent of the time. The beauty of this rule is that you have the freedom to interpret it in your own way. For example, you can choose to have 80 percent healthy and 20 percent less healthy foods per meal, or you can eat healthy 80 percent of the week and allow yourself some indulgence for the remaining 20 percent.

This approach allows you to maintain a good balance without imposing strict rules on yourself. You can continue to enjoy your meals while avoiding excessive indulgence.

LIFE IS SHORT, TREAT YOURSELF.

Be kind.

That's the danger of diets: they are difficult or impossible to sustain. The 80/20 rule can also be applied to alcohol consumption. Don't drink too much or too often; choose your moments. For example, save it for a fun weekend evening instead of opening a bottle of wine every weeknight. Because at that point, do you even notice it anymore? Are you still enjoying it? Or has it just become a bad habit? How do you feel after a night of drinking? When you're back on track and in a healthy flow, it often feels amazing. And who wouldn't want that?

To do: Plan your meals according to the 80/20 rule.

Try to schedule your meals as best as possible in your week using the 80/20 rule. This way, you won't be caught off guard, skipping meals, or reaching for unhealthy options when you lack inspiration. You've already planned it out for yourself!

Note: If you feel that your body needs something different, that's perfectly okay! Again, don't be too hard on yourself.

MONDAY

TUESDAY

WEDNESDAY

THURSDAY

FRIDAY

SATURDAY

SUNDAY

It is also helpful to schedule a moment in the week for grocery shopping. Whether you do it in a physical store or online, take a moment to calmly think about what you need, so you don't make impulsive decisions. It starts with creating a shopping list. If meal planning is still a challenge, you can simply stock up on plenty of healthy items that can be used to prepare various delicious and nutritious meals.

For example, lettuce, tuna, avocado, tomatoes, granola, plant-based yogurt, lots of vegetables and fruits, and tasty crackers. Having a basic shopping list of healthy and delicious items is very convenient. Once I have all the products at home on Monday and my fridge looks full and especially healthy, it instantly makes me happy. Then my week can begin!

To do: Buy basic groceries.

Create your basic grocery list with products that you can use for breakfast, lunch, dinner, and snacks. Maybe you already have some items you buy every week? Put the list on your phone or on a paper you can put in your shopping bag. This way, you'll never get lost in the supermarket again!

_____   _____
_____   _____
_____   _____
_____   _____
_____   _____
_____   _____
_____   _____

Every day, your beautiful body is doing its best for you. We often take for granted that our body functions well until something goes wrong, and then we have a so-called "wake-up call." It's usually after that moment that we start to appreciate our bodies. Be aware of all the things your body does for you and reward it by nourishing it with enough nutrients.

Eating should remain enjoyable, and it's important that you also find it delicious and not eat just because you have to. Have fun with recipes, make lists for yourself, and go out for meals when you have the opportunity. Don't take it too seriously and don't punish yourself if you've "indulged" too much. Our bodies need fuel, and it's good to consider what exactly your body needs. Just don't let it become an obsession. Trust your intuition, eat when you're hungry, and don't when you're not hungry. Consume plenty of vitamins because they give you energy and savor those moments when you deviate from your usual routine. When you eat well, you feel better because you're happy that you're nourishing yourself. Remember that! After all, you're doing it for yourself because you are important.

Exercise

Our bodies need maintenance too. It's important that we pay attention to it. Just like nutrition, our bodies need exercise to keep all the muscles and joints supple. In addition, regular physical activity puts your heart and blood vessels to work, making them stronger and keeping your veins healthy. Exercise improves blood flow to the brain, which has a very positive impact on your mood, immune system, and stress reduction. Since we spend so much time sitting, we need to keep moving to function properly. In the Western world, we have created our own pitfalls by providing ourselves with so much convenience. The paradox is that we spoil our bodies too much and make it too easy for our muscles and joints. Our joints and muscles need to be well circulated, and you can achieve that by engaging in sports. All types of sports are good: tennis, football, hockey, yoga, dancing, and so on.

Do what you enjoy and what makes you happy!

To do: How do you exercise?

Sports I did as a child:

Sports in which I feel confident:

Sports that help me relax:

During these sports, I have the most fun:

_____
_____
_____
_____
_____

Sports I want to try:

_____
_____
_____
_____
_____

Staying flexible and stretching is good for us, otherwise, we'll become stiff. When something is stuck, it breaks. By moving your body and putting pressure on it, you keep it healthy. The beauty is that we can all do this, and everyone can do it in their own way. For example, you can start by sitting on the floor in a cross-legged position instead of on a chair.

Personally, I find animal flows very enjoyable and beneficial. You can do them at home at a time of your choosing. They make you flexible and strong, and being close to the ground helps you feel connected to nature. It can be challenging at first, but you'll quickly get used to it. Everyone can do it at their own pace.

There are also many yoga flows available online that are very good for you. It's your choice not to stay on the couch but to get moving. By doing this, you send yourself a signal that you are important. You take care of yourself.

**Move,
love,
flow,
change,
grow,
power,
grit,
strength.**

The best feeling is when you can exercise outdoors. You feel doubly fit afterward. It gives you so much energy because you're getting extra oxygen. Nature heals you. It's good to incorporate outdoor exercise into your new lifestyle. Plan it, find a routine, and above all, stick with it.

If you take a break, it's okay! Just start again when you find the strength. Nobody is always motivated; you have to rely on perseverance. Do you have that in you?

To do: Fitness goals.

How often do you want to exercise per week?

_____
_____
_____
_____
_____
_____

What do you want to achieve? (Flexibility, strength, endurance, etc.)

_____
_____
_____
_____
_____

How fit/flexible do you want to be?

_____
_____
_____
_____
_____

Sometimes you may not have the strength to go to the gym or attend team sports training. That's okay. But consider what kind of person you are when choosing your sport(s). Can you motivate yourself well? Then an individual sport is handy. Do you perform better with teammates? Then a team sport is more suitable for you. Try to figure this out for yourself. Do you need someone to do it with? Are you someone who cancels easily? If your friend cancels, do you also not go? Sometimes it's okay not to go. But try not to just lie on the couch!

Exercise can be intense, but movement is something you do every day. Find movement in the small daily things. Take the bike instead of the car, take the stairs instead of the elevator, and go to the store instead of placing an order.

To do: How fit do you want to feel? How flexible do you want to be?

For example, going to the beach with the dog, going to the gym with a friend, etc.

_____
_____
_____
_____
_____
_____
_____
_____
_____
_____
_____
_____
_____

"It never gets easier, you just get better"

You'll feel better once you've done it, even if you didn't feel like it at first. Exercise is good for you and gives you energy, especially when done outdoors! Find consistency in your physical activities and engage in sports that you enjoy. Explore what fits into your schedule and play around with it. For example, try exercising before going to work/school. You can also exercise on your own mat at home!

Consider your goals regarding physical activity and how you feel in your body. How do you want to feel in a few months? How do you want to see yourself in the mirror? Always listen to your body and what it needs.

Don't overdo it, don't go to extremes, but definitely keep going!

Me-time

Me-time: What is "me-time"? And why do we actually need it? Me-time is time that is completely, 100 percent, our own, time that you can dedicate entirely to yourself, filling it in the way you want. It's time you don't have to be accountable to anyone, not even to yourself. Does me-time have to be alone time? No, it doesn't have to be. You can also spend it with someone who brings you joy. However, you should genuinely want this and not do it because you think someone else wants it. After all, it's your time, and you should fill it the way you want.

Finding a good balance between work, leisure, family, and other aspects of life is important. We often put too much pressure on ourselves, which leads to stress and sometimes even results in burnout. To ensure that you are in balance and feel good, there are a few important things, such as nutrition, exercise, and of course, me-time.

I hope you can find a beautiful balance between what you have to do and what you truly want, and that you start seeing things like exercise, nutrition, and me-time as important. Become aware of the time you have and learn to let go of unimportant matters so that you have more time for yourself. Because you are important. Regularly schedule time for yourself without feeling guilty about it. You will feel so much better when you allow yourself to prioritize time for yourself, to give yourself that gift, and truly enjoy it. Why should someone or something else be more important than you? After all, you have control over your own life.

To do: Your ultimate me-time moments.

When I have a me-time afternoon, evening, or day, it often looks like this:

_____
_____
_____
_____
_____

I prefer to spend a me-time moment like this:

_____
_____
_____
_____

Me-time ideas:

✦ *Take a walk while listening to a pleasant podcast or your favorite music.*
✦ *Read a nice magazine or a few pages from a beautiful book.*
✦ *Go on a shopping spree: online or in the city!*
✦ *Practice yoga or meditation.*
✦ *Clean up: An organized space is an organized mind.*
✦ *Cook or bake something elaborate.*
✦ *Social media detox.*
✦ *Get artsy! Drawing, painting, etc.*
✦ *Plan your next vacation/trip.*
✦ *Write in your journal. ;)*
✦ *Create a detailed plan or to-do list.*

Me-time is about choosing yourself, being present and in the moment, and giving attention to yourself. Anything you give attention to becomes more beautiful. Take some time to explore what brings you joy and happiness. Baking a cake, going to the hairdresser, applying a face mask, exercising, taking a bath, reading a book, sleeping in, working in the garden, tidying up, organizing closets, buying and filling in a new planner, and so on!

Me-time = YOU time!

During me-time, you are processing and recovering from all the stimuli you receive throughout the day. During me-time, be in the moment and try not to spend too much time on your phone. Some people need more alone time than others, but me-time can also be spent with someone else.

Call a friend with whom you can do something fun. Go to the movies, have dinner, take a walk, or exercise together. Engage in meaningful conversations and listen to each other's stories, so you can learn from one another. Most importantly, enjoy each other's company and have a great time together.

Note: Are you afraid of being alone with your thoughts? Sometimes, that can be scary. However, it is even more unpleasant to make plans with people you don't really want to be with just because you fear being alone or because you experience FOMO (Fear of Missing Out). Be careful not to surround yourself with people solely because you associate being alone with something negative. Being alone can bring beautiful things and provide perspective. Find a good balance in this.

If you notice that you feel dull or not fully present in a social setting, that's probably a signal to take a step back and take more time for yourself.

To do: Schedule your me-time.

Schedule at least two me-time moments in the planner on the following page. Consider what you will do, whether it's alone or with someone else, and when. Listen to yourself carefully. Would you prefer to do this in your own agenda or planner? That's fine too! As long as you have visibility and awareness of it.

MONDAY

TUESDAY

WEDNESDAY

THURSDAY

FRIDAY

SATURDAY

SUNDAY

In part 2, you created a "Happy List." These are things you can incorporate into your me-time moments. Discover what you need at different times, whether it's spending time alone or with someone else. Being comfortable with being alone is not an art, but it may take some practice for some people. Dare to be alone and do what you feel like doing. Not having to consider others can be delightful at times.

Ask yourself what you want. Being comfortable with being alone is not hard, as long as you simply do what you feel like doing. So, be yourself and enjoy your own company. Be able to be alone and embrace it. Self-care and me-time look different for everyone, so find the routine that works for you!

Today I choose me

Taking time for yourself sometimes means disappointing people. In other words, standing up for yourself. Saying yes or no to something can be difficult. However, once you start practicing it, you'll notice that you quickly get the hang of it and feel proud of yourself. You can practice this at home, with friends, parents, at school, at work, or even in a restaurant. Being able to say no is part of it. Why should something come at your expense? You now know who you are, what you want, and what you stand for: dare to prioritize yourself.

Stop pleasing others, which means doing things just to make someone else happy. The attention you normally give to others now goes to yourself. You are simply worth it. Why should someone else be more important? You will determine how you want to be treated, and you need to take responsibility for it yourself. That way, you can never blame someone else.

Have you ever thought about who is actually to blame for how you feel? Do you often blame something or someone else?

Things always happen in your life, both good and not so good. It's how you deal with them that determines how you feel. Who do you blame for your "misfortune"? Do you blame yourself? Or do you take responsibility? Look for answers within yourself when you blame something or someone for a situation. It's time to stand up for yourself and take control of your life.

"The power is in your own hands."

To do: Practice standing up for yourself.

How do I react when someone asks me for something I don't have time for?
___
___

How do I react when someone asks me to do something I don't feel like doing?
___
___

How do I react when someone asks me about something I don't support?
_____
_____
_____

How do I react when someone makes a nasty comment about me?
_____
_____
_____

How do I react when someone takes me for granted?
_____
_____
_____

How do I react when someone speaks for me?
_____
_____
_____

Facing Fears

Taking care of yourself also means doing things that you dread, don't want to do, or are afraid to do. These can be divided into laziness and fear. Are you too lazy to do something? Or are you genuinely afraid that you can't do it?

To do: Create a to-do list with tasks you have been dreading for a while.

Think of administrative tasks or that annoying chore at home. When are you going to do this? Consider doing one task per week, depending on how time-consuming the task is, or maybe even two! Put it in your calendar if necessary. Bet you'll feel good once it's done!

TO DO:

Apart from things you don't feel like doing, there may also be things you want to do but are afraid to do. You may be afraid of failure or afraid that something might happen to you or someone else. But deep down, there is always a flicker of desire for something you truly want.

So why not go for it? A big part of taking care of yourself is stepping out of your comfort zone. Doing things that genuinely make you happy. Think about that one thing you've always wanted to do. How proud would you be if you actually did it? Can you feel the excitement building up? Realize that fear is nothing more than a thought followed by a feeling.

A thought is not the truth or the reality. You can breathe through it when something feels scary, and you'll see that nothing terrible happens. You can do it. Maybe not the first time or the next time, but eventually, you will. By facing these fears, your insecurity transforms into self-assurance. See, you are capable of doing it, aren't you?

To do: Face your fears.

What would you do if fear wasn't an issue?

_____
_____
_____

What could happen that you're so afraid of? Worst-case scenario?

_____
_____
_____

Is this a realistic fear?

_____
_____
_____

What do you need to do to set aside this fear? Do you need any help with it?

_____
_____
_____

What is the best-case scenario? What if nothing goes wrong?

_____
_____
_____

How will you overcome this fear?

_____
_____
_____

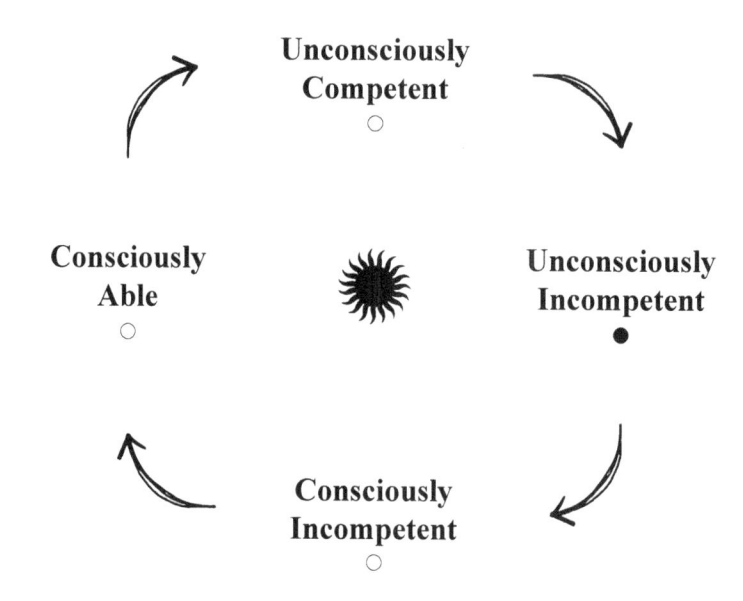

Unconsciously Competent
○

Unconsciously Incompetent
●

Consciously Incompetent
○

Consciously Able
○

Yes! You are now "consciously competent"! You know who you are, what you want and can do, and how to take care of yourself. The only thing that needs to happen now is to take action, which might be the most challenging part. You have all the knowledge and motivation, but how do you persevere? The good news is that if you persist and show discipline for a while, it will eventually become natural. You have organized your life in such a way that achieving what you want almost happens effortlessly because you no longer have to think about it. You are then "unconsciously competent."

In part 4, we will teach you how to become fully "unconsciously competent." You will design your mind in a way that you believe you can achieve anything you set your mind to. Everything you have thought about during the journaling process will be transformed into actions that eventually become habits.

To do: Summarize of part 3.

After part 3, I know why it is important to take care of myself, namely:

_____
_____
_____
_____
_____

After part 3, I know what I need to do to take better care of myself, namely:

_____
_____
_____
_____
_____

After part 3, I know how I am going to take care of myself, namely:

_____
_____
_____
_____
_____

After part 3, I feel:

_____
_____
_____
_____
_____

You have completed part 3, well done! Do you now understand why it's important to take good care of yourself? And that anything that receives time and attention will grow? The most important, but perhaps also the most challenging, aspect of part 3 is listening to your body. What do you need at any given moment? Try practicing this. If you find yourself feeling tired for several consecutive days and don't know why, something may have gone wrong in taking care of yourself. Try to prevent this! You don't want to start eating healthy only when you get sick, and you don't want to get a good night's sleep only after staying up for multiple nights.

At some point, you will better understand what your body needs, have more energy, and feel better overall. You'll know who you are, be open to change, and know what you need to achieve that. I am already so proud of you for making it this far. You can be proud of yourself, you deserve it!

REPEAT AFTER ME:

- *I am worthy of being cared for.*
- *I deserve time for myself.*
- *I love good food and will continue to enjoy it.*
- *I enjoy moving my body with ease.*
- *My body takes me where I need to be.*
- *I can stand up for myself.*
- *I dare to set my boundaries.*
- *I dare to face my fears.*
- *I do everything in due time and at my own pace.*
- *I am proud of myself.*
- *I love who I am and want to take care of myself.*
- *I care for myself as I would care for loved ones.*
- *I believe in myself.*

Which emotions do you feel after part 3?
Circle, cross out, highlight, or add the ones that apply to you.

Motivated

Strong

Positive

CONFIDENT

Energetic

RELIEVED

Proud

Touched

Happy

EMOTIONAL

Sad

Room for thought

✧ *Gratitude* ✧

Three things I am grateful for:

_____
_____
_____
_____

Three things I am looking forward to or that were fun today:

_____
_____
_____
_____

Three positive affirmations:

_____
_____
_____
_____

Rate your mood

☆ ☆ ☆ ☆ ☆

✧ *Gratitude* ✧

Three things I am grateful for:

___
___
___

Three things I am looking forward to or that were fun today:

___
___
___

Three positive affirmations:

___
___
___

Rate your mood

☆ ☆ ☆ ☆ ☆

✧ *Gratitude* ✧

Three things I am grateful for:

_____
_____
_____

Three things I am looking forward to or that were fun today:

_____
_____
_____

Three positive affirmations:

_____
_____
_____

Rate your mood

☆ ☆ ☆ ☆ ☆

Part 4

The Plan

~ ***The plan...*** The world lies at our feet, and life is too short not to fully enjoy it. I hope I have inspired you so far to take good care of yourself, to move, and stand up for yourself. I hope you realize how much naturally falls into place when you make choices from the heart and understand that you have control over your thoughts. I want to convey to you what positive energy can bring and that you can achieve anything as long as you set your mind to it.

It's all in the mindset!

If you think you can do something, you can. Believe in yourself, be kind to yourself, and persevere. In part 1, you learned that you have influence over your own thoughts. How will you make this work in your favor when it comes to achieving your goals?

To do: Master your thoughts.

How will you take control of your thoughts?

_____
_____
_____
_____

What will you do when negative thoughts take over?

_____
_____
_____
_____

How do you want to think about yourself and your life? What is your goal?

_____
_____
_____
_____

☾

You have influence over what you think and, as a result, you can adjust your choices accordingly. In this way, you can determine what your life looks like. After all, you have control over how you handle an event and whether you focus on the positive or the negative. It's a perspective, an insight. You choose to pay attention to things you have influence over and let go of things you have no control over.

To do: Master your thoughts 2.0.

When I have insecure thoughts about myself, I choose to exchange these thoughts for:

_____
_____
_____
_____
_____

When I have the idea that I can't do something, I give myself confidence by thinking that:

_____
_____
_____

When I have too many thoughts that lead to overthinking and rumination, I solve that by:

_____
_____
_____

When I find myself comparing myself too much to others in my mind, I stop that by:

_____
_____
_____

Through our life experiences, we have created beliefs about ourselves. When you start working on them, you realize that the voices in your head are just thoughts. You learn to recognize them. Examples of these voices are the perfectionist, the helper, the professional, the controller, the pusher, the critic, the learner, the independent one, the insecure one, and the tough one. It's up to you how you deal with them.

We can use the BUS method; you have control over which voice you put at the wheel of your bus. If you let the negative voice take over, there is less space for positive thoughts.

Once you become aware of this and follow your intuition, peace and balance arise. You start living by your own intuition and listening to what your heart desires. We often already know it, but we don't listen to it.

To do: The bus.

Who do you put at the wheel? Who are the passengers on the bus? Do you remember when you started this journal, did you have a goal? Did you want to feel more confident? Did you want to please less and stand up for yourself more? Or did you want to think less and do more?

This is the moment to apply that. What is most important to you? Which voice do you put at the front of the bus? Which passengers are allowed on the journey? And more importantly, who do you leave behind?

On the next page, write down who you put behind the wheel and who else is on the bus.

Who's in control?

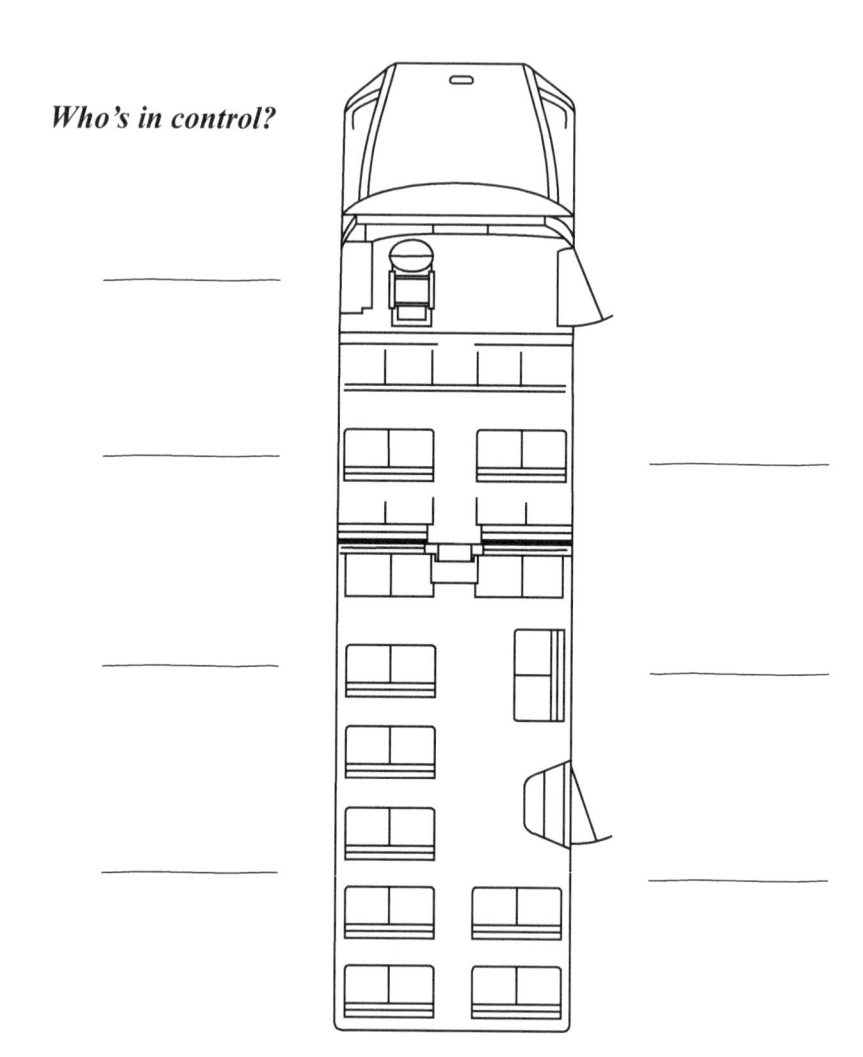

I would write down at the beginning: self-confidence. The thoughts I want to bring along are gratitude and determination. Thoughts I want to leave behind are perfectionism, excessive worrying, and jealousy toward others. How about you?

I strongly believe that you need to make a plan and set goals for yourself. You now know what your pitfalls are and can take them into account when planning. For example, if you struggle with exercising in the morning, schedule it in the evening! If your goal is to be a morning person but you always go to bed late, take action!

Once you have written out a plan and visualized it for yourself, it becomes easier to reach your goal. Ask yourself: Do I really want this? If the answer is yes, go for it! Of course, there are always exceptions and things may not go as planned. In those moments, take a break. Everyone needs a different approach, and you are the only one who knows what that is. It's a matter of finding balance between challenging yourself and being kind to yourself. Look in the mirror each time and ask yourself, "Am I doing well?" Be honest with yourself. If not, give yourself a kick in the butt, but also give yourself a compliment right away. The most important thing is that you make progress, and you should be proud of that.

You're doing great, you go! We will delve deeper into setting life goals in the short and long term shortly.

To do: Creating habits.

In part 1: "Believing in Change," you identified the general beliefs about yourself and your life that you want to change. Now we will translate those into concrete actions.

What are specific things you want to change about yourself and your life? For example, I want to exercise at least two times a week, I want to drink two liters of water per day, and I want to meet up with a friend every weekend.

_____
_____
_____
_____
_____
_____
_____
_____

Creating habits is essential for achieving your goals and changing your life. When something becomes a habit, you do it without thinking about it. You do it now, for example, while brushing your teeth, taking a shower, or performing any other activity that comes naturally. But it also applies to things like scrolling on your phone for hours, lounging on the couch every evening, or eating unhealthy food. These may be less desirable habits, but because you are so used to them, you don't consider them as something you can or want to change.

Now, imagine that the goals you wrote above become habits that you do every day, without thinking about it. How wonderful would that be? It does require some effort at the beginning. You have to do it repeatedly and push yourself to keep doing it. Then, the rule applies that everything becomes familiar.

If nothing changes, nothing changes.

Read that again.

If you don't start changing something, nothing will happen.

To do: Plan.

Create a schedule for this week. Realize that if you don't put things in the schedule, there's a good chance you won't do them. Refer back to the specific goals you set earlier in your journal. For example, if you want to exercise twice a week, schedule it for times when you actually have the time and energy to do it. Consider every part you have been working on so far: schedule "me-time," exercise, grocery shopping, work, leisure activities, administrative tasks, cooking, laundry, etc. Make sure not to overbook your weekend. If you complete all your tasks this week, it will be easier to do them again next week! Create a routine that brings you joy. This way, you'll shift from a fixed mindset to a growth mindset. You are growing and achieving your goals.

Tip: Rewrite it in your own agenda or planner if it helps you.

MONDAY

TUESDAY

WEDNESDAY

THURSDAY

FRIDAY

SATURDAY

SUNDAY

What you have just done is create a weekly schedule. These are the things you want to do. How does it feel? To have the sense that you're working toward something? Having goals in life is essential. How would you structure your life so that you become the best version of yourself? You will lead a life that aligns perfectly with who you are and fulfills your dreams—dream big! The beautiful thing is that once you have a plan, everything becomes clearer, and you gradually get used to the idea. Imagine if it were to succeed. How would you feel?

Let's do that. Let's go!

To do: Set dreams, goals, and ambitions.

We start by writing down our dreams, goals, and ambitions.

_____
_____
_____
_____
_____

To get there, you need both a plan for the upcoming year, as well as for the long term. It's important that your various dreams, goals, and ambitions align with each other so that they contribute to achieving your ultimate goals. For example, if your goal is to see as much of the world as possible, that's great! But it's quite broad. Your short-term goal that can contribute to this is, for instance, taking a beautiful trip this year and going on three trips within the next three years. That's achievable, right? Realize that you can't do everything at once. Focus on the things that truly matter to you, and that's when you're most likely to succeed!

To do: Set short-term goals.

WHAT DO YOU WANT TO HAVE ACHIEVED IN ONE YEAR?

How do I want to feel:

_____
_____
_____

I have left behind these emotions:

_____
_____
_____

Any other goals? Personal or professional. Write them down!

_____
_____
_____
_____
_____
_____

WHAT DO YOU WANT TO HAVE ACHIEVED IN FIVE YEARS?

How do I want to feel:

___

I have left behind these emotions:

___

Any other goals? Personal or professional. Write them down!

___

Does life control you or do YOU control life?

You have now created your dreams, goals, and ambitions. Just by looking at them, you should feel happy. You are going to do something you've always wanted to do, something you may not yet believe you can actually achieve. There may be a voice in your head saying, "You can't do that," or "You're too scared." But now you know that these thoughts are not true. Think of the bus and make sure you put the right person behind the wheel. That way, you start thinking in terms of possibilities. You are worthy, and you are going to fight for it. Is it difficult? Yes, sometimes it is. But you persevere and keep your focus. Once you start believing in yourself, you will realize that the possibilities are endless.

You can do this!

You now know yourself much better and what you need. You take care of yourself and stand up for yourself. With this final step, you will finally believe in something you never thought possible for yourself. You are worth so much more than you used to think, and you should be proud of that.

Now you're going to turn your dreams, goals, and ambitions into action. It's time to make them concrete.

To do: Make dreams concrete.

During part 2, you described your dream life and wrote down your dreams, goals, and ambitions for the medium and long term. How are you going to make them happen? For example, I want to take a solo trip to a distant destination. I will save money, book the trip, and not let the fear of feeling alone hold me back. In fact, I will be very proud of myself and learn a lot from the experience!

I want to:

_____
_____
_____

So I will:

_____
_____
_____

I want to:

___
___
___

So I will:

___
___
___

✧

I want to:

___
___
___

So I will:

___
___
___

I want to:

So I will:

✧

I want to:

So I will:

I want to:

So I will:

✧

I want to:

So I will:

To do: Life goals.

This is how I want to approach life:

_____
_____
_____

This is how I want to be remembered:

_____
_____
_____

This is how I want to think about myself:

_____
_____
_____

This is how I want others to see me:

_____
_____
_____
_____
_____
_____

This is how I want to leave the world:

_____
_____
_____
_____
_____
_____

Many of the goals you set can be achieved through routine. Once you have a routine, you perform these actions without thinking about them. You are unconsciously competent! By building a good and healthy routine, you can structure it in a way that brings you closer to your goals. For example, if you want more energy, it starts at the beginning of your day. Wake up early, exercise, and have breakfast (which can also be at eleven or noon if you practice intermittent fasting). Do you struggle to wake up in the morning? Taking a cold shower can work wonders! It may take some getting used to at first, but eventually, it becomes natural. Create a routine that suits you.

If you fall out of your routine, it's okay! Be kind to yourself and get back on track quickly. It's normal for routines to be different when you go on vacation or find yourself in a different setting.

Although your environment influences your routines to some extent, you have a significant amount of control over them. The better you stick to your routines, the easier everything becomes.

To do: Establish routines.

MY MORNING ROUTINE

7:00	
8:00	
9:00	
10:00	
11:00	
12:00	
13:00	

MY EVENING ROUTINE

16:00

17:00

18:00

19:00

20:00

21:00

22:00

MY WEEKEND ROUTINE

10:00	_____
11:00	_____
12:00	_____
13:00	_____
14:00	_____
15:00	_____
16:00	_____
17:00	_____
18:00	_____
19:00	_____
20:00	_____
21:00	_____

RESPONSIBILITY SHOULD BE IN NO ONE'S HANDS BUT YOUR OWN.

Don't make excuses based on events in your life to not stick to your plan. Things will always happen; life is shaped by situations. But you determine how you deal with situations. That determines how you will feel. Will you give up? Will you throw away your goals and routines? Of course not! You will keep going because every situation can be put into perspective. In certain situations, your body and mind may need different things than usual, for example, when going through a sad period. Even then, you have the choice of how to handle the situation. Allow yourself to truly feel sad, take time for it, and pick up the pieces when it feels right for you. Never suppress sadness, tears need to be shed, it heals you.

Don't blame others either, life is sometimes unfair. You are responsible for your own happiness. Keep your goal in mind and learn to prioritize. If you really listen to your intuition, you will know where your priorities lie, and you will organize your time in a way that brings you closer to your goal. That's what you want, that's what you promised yourself, and you can do it!

You have completed part 4, and I am so proud of you! Are you proud of yourself too? That's great! The essence of part 4 is that you are in charge of your own mind. You have the choice of what to think and you can do anything you want if you believe you can. In other words, it's about believing in yourself. Because if you don't believe in yourself, who will? You are worth believing in. You now know what you want to achieve and how you're going to do it. I hope this gives you a new sense of vitality and energy you may have lost but have now found again. You feel better because you're making good choices, taking responsibility for your own life, and taking care of yourself. If you keep doing this long enough, you'll notice that it becomes natural. The negative thoughts that try to bring you down will diminish and eventually disappear! How amazing is that? At that moment, you will officially be unconsciously competent. You decide!

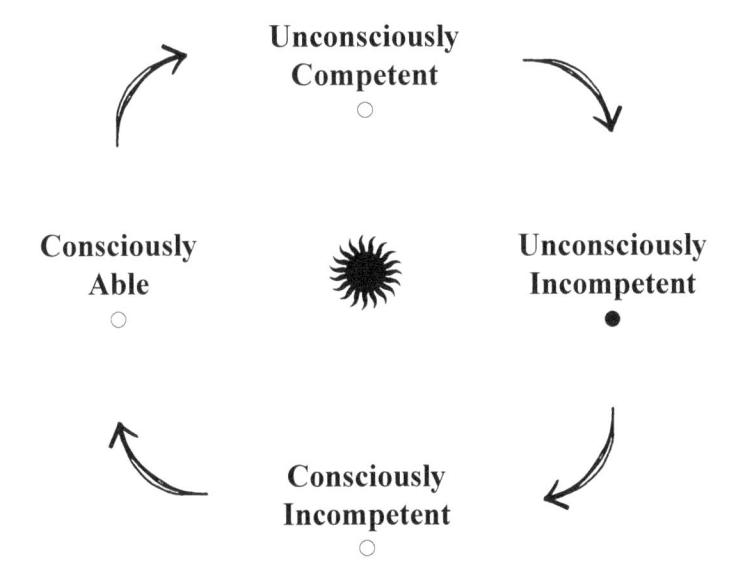

Unconsciously Competent

Consciously Able

Unconsciously Incompetent

Consciously Incompetent

To do: Summarize part 4.

After part 4, I feel:

REPEAT AFTER ME:

- *I know what I want in this life.*
- *I know exactly what I need to do to get where I want to be.*
- *I will push myself to be the best version of myself.*
- *I make the right choices in dealing with situations.*
- *I won't dwell on setbacks when things get tough.*
- *I know where my priorities lie.*
- *I dare to dream big.*
- *I have control over my thoughts.*
- *I believe in myself.*
- *I know I can do anything by believing I can.*
- *I am proud of who I am.*
- *I continue to challenge and develop myself.*
- *I am willing to help others with my knowledge.*
- *I am happy.*

☾

START MAKING YOUR OWN MANUAL.

Create your dream life.

Which emotions do you feel after part 4?
Circle, underline, highlight, or add the ones that apply to you.

Motivated

Strong

_____

Positive

CONFIDENT

_____

Active

RELIEVED

Proud

Touched

Happy

EMOTIONAL

Sad

Room for thought

✦ Gratitude ✦

Three things I am grateful for:

_____
_____
_____
_____

Three things I am looking forward to or that were fun today:

_____
_____
_____
_____

Three positive affirmations:

_____
_____
_____
_____

Rate your mood

☆ ☆ ☆ ☆ ☆

✧ *Gratitude* ✧

Three things I am grateful for:

_____
_____
_____

Three things I am looking forward to or that were fun today:

_____
_____
_____

Three positive affirmations:

_____
_____
_____

Rate your mood

☆ ☆ ☆ ☆ ☆

✧ *Gratitude* ✧

Three things I am grateful for:

_____
_____
_____

Three things I am looking forward to or that were fun today:

_____
_____
_____

Three positive affirmations:

_____
_____
_____

Rate your mood

☆ ☆ ☆ ☆ ☆

Be proud of you!

You have completed this journal! You did it. By finishing it, you have given yourself something truly special. Every time you worked on it, you invested in yourself, and that is a significant step. You should be proud because it is even bigger than you realize. The mindset of possibilities, and the desire to learn, grow, and improve is so cool. This is just the beginning!

You have laid the foundation of awareness, and I hope a whole new world has opened up for you, making things clearer. We can achieve so much more than we think!

I hope I have inspired you to do things differently, things that align more with who you are. To seek out a new, wonderful, unique, and beautiful version of yourself.

A NOTE FROM MAGGIE

Make my Way, your Way. It's so amazing to see that we are all different, and you can create your own user manual. You now know that you have choices, goals, and dreams. If you start believing in them and make them come true, wow, how cool is that? You know my motto: DARE TO BE.

I am so proud of everyone who has purchased this book because you already knew that there was more inside you than was coming out. Now you are really starting to realize it. Take the time to process this journey and enjoy it. Sometimes it goes fast, and sometimes it goes slow, but they are all phases. You are already an expert, in a way.

As you know, I love sharing and passing things on. How amazing would it be if you could contribute to that by telling people about this book? So that they can also grow and become better. Let others experience this too!

I understand if you have questions or even the need for a conversation. Let me know if there's anything I can do for you. I'm here for you!

Love,

Maggie

BOOK LIST

Tuesdays with Morrie by Mitch Albom
A Different View on Giftedness by Marike Althuizen, Esther de Boer, and Nathalie Kordelaar
Gifted by Tessa Kieboom
Happiness Advantage by Shawn Achor
Highly Sensitive Persons by Elaine N. Aron
Daring Greatly by Brené Brown
Vulnerability by Brené Brown
Humankind: A Hopeful History by Rutger Bregman
Mindset by Carol S. Dweck
Ikigai by Francesc Miralles and Hector Garcia
Wabi Sabi by Beth Kempton
Restart by Rogier van Kralingen
*The Subtle Art of Not Giving a F*ck* by Mark Manson
The Miracle of Water by Dr. Masaru Emoto
How to Change by Katy Milkman
The Chimp Paradox by Dr. Steve Peters
No Bad Parts by Richard Schwartz
The Things You Can See Only When You Slow Down by Haemin Sunim
Surrender to Your Adversity by Rob Swymer
Woman by Lucy Woesthoff
Sick Happy by Ruud ten Wolde

Dream it. Wish it. Do it

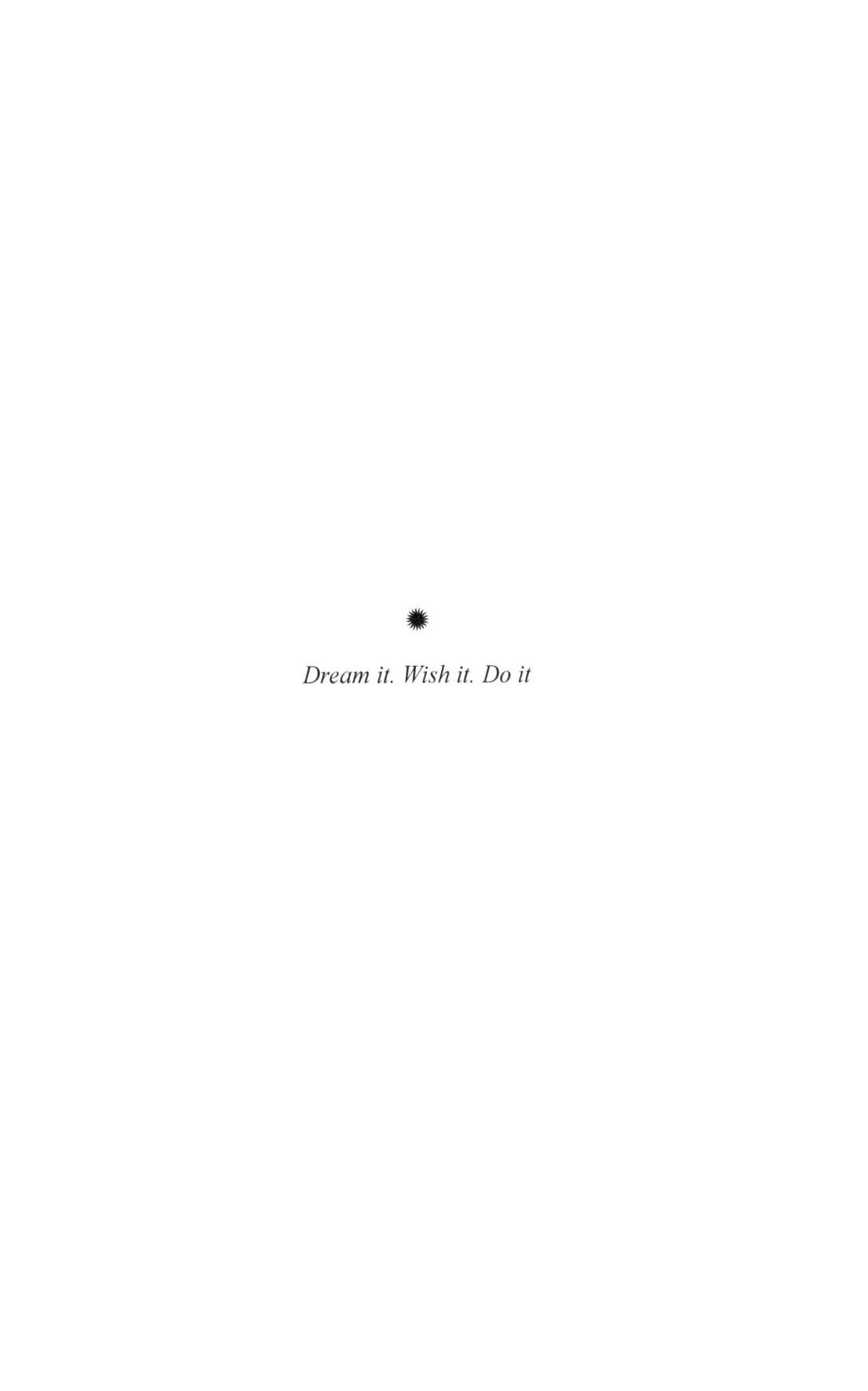

GET IN TOUCH

*Let me know if there's anything I can do for you.
I'm here for you!*

WWW.MAGGIESWAY.NL   @MAGGIES WAY

HERE YOU CAN MAKE THE TEST FOR HSP

NEED MORE ?

*To further assist you in this beautiful process, there are so many possibilities.
Here are three that can help you fully connect with yourself.*

TIME TO REFLECT

Mandali Retreat
Italy

Zest for Life
Turkey

Yoga retreats
Worldwide

*You can also always call your general practitioner, and in case of emergency, call 911,
or for Suicide and Crisis lifeline, call 988.*

ACKNOWLEDGMENTS

In the journey of crafting this book, I am eternally grateful for the unwavering love and support that my family has shown me. Your encouragement has been my guiding light, for always being so proud of me, and illuminating even in the most challenging of writing days. Thank you for your patience and always believing in me. You all are my inspiration every day.

To my children, I am very grateful to say that, despite all the challenges and difficult times, you have blossomed into remarkable, amazing, and beautiful individuals, both inside and out.

I also want to express my gratitude and thanks to all those who played a role in transforming this idea into reality. Your dedication, insight, and collaborative spirit have added depth and richness to each chapter. This journey would not have been the same without your contributions.

And to you, the readers, I offer my sincerest hope. May these words resonate with your experiences, dreams, and aspirations. In the pages of this book, I wish for you to find reflections of yourself, and may it guide you toward the pathway of self-discovery and happiness so you can live the life you have always dreamed of—because you are worth it.

With love,

Maggie

Milton Keynes UK
Ingram Content Group UK Ltd.
UKHW021143100324
438949UK00002B/5